JOHN PARRILLO'S
50
WORKOUT
SECRETS

JOHN PARRILLO'S 50 WORKOUT SECRETS

John Parrillo
and Maggie Greenwood-Robinson

A Perigee Book

A Perigee Book
Published by The Berkley Publishing Group
200 Madison Avenue
New York, NY 10016

Book design by James McGuire
Front and back cover photos © 1994 by Ralph DeHaan
Cover model: Dennis Newman
Photograph of John Parrillo © 1994 by Barry Brooks
Cover design by Andrew M. Newman

Individual dietary needs vary, and no one diet will meet everyone's
requirements. Before beginning any diet or exercise program, consult your
physician. Do not take nutritional supplements without your physician's
approval. Responsibility for any adverse effects or unforeseen consequences
resulting from the use of the information contained herein is expressly
disclaimed.

Library of Congress Cataloging-in-Publication Data
Parrillo, John.
    [50 workout secrets]
    John Parrillo's 50 workout secrets / by John Parrillo and Maggie Greenwood-Robinson.
        p. cm.
    ISBN 0–399–51862–2
    1. Bodybuilding—Training.   2. Athletes—Nutrition.
    I. Greenwood-Robinson, Maggie.   II. Title: III. Title: 50 workout secrets.   IV. Title: Fifty workout secrets.
    GV546.5.P365   1994
    646.7′5—dc20   94–1607
                                                                                        CIP

Printed in the United States of America
10 9 8 7 6 5 4 3 2 1

Contents

Acknowledgments

It is exciting to see this second book published, and there are many people to thank for its production:

All the amateur and professional bodybuilders and athletes with whom I've worked—especially Dennis Newman.

Maggie Greenwood-Robinson, my coauthor, who has worked with me for five years now. Maggie crafted my 50 nutrition and training secrets into a fine text, worked with several well-known photographers, and organized the best of their work into this book.

Robert Kennedy, publisher of *MuscleMag International*. Bob continues to support me by publishing my "Parrillo Performance" column in his successful magazine and promoting my work whenever he can. Bob is a great friend as well.

Greg Zulak, one of the finest bodybuilding journalists I have ever known. Through his articles, Greg has been instrumental in getting the Parrillo message out to millions of readers.

Lou Zwick, producer and creator of *American Muscle Magazine*, seen on ESPN. Lou has graciously promoted the Parrillo Performance programs on his show, including an excellent feature on my first book, *High Performance Bodybuilding*.

John Balik, publisher of *Ironman Magazine*. John has taken a sincere interest in my nutrition and training techniques and has gone to great lengths to help me promote many of my programs.

Rochelle Larkin, editor of *Female Bodybuilding*. Rochelle is another one of my "advocates" and favorite people. She believes in what we are doing at Parrillo Performance and helps spread the word to others.

Steve Wennerstrom of *Women's Physique World*. Steve has been supportive by publicizing our programs in his magazines and contributing to our own magazine, *John Parrillo's Performance Press*.

Cliff Sheats, clinical nutritionist. Cliff has been an inspiration and a great help in promoting our products and methods to a large audience of fitness enthusiasts.

Joe Weider, publisher of *Muscle & Fitness*, FLEX, *Shape*, and other leading fitness magazines. Joe single-handedly made bodybuilding the popular fitness pursuit it is today, inspiring others to become the best they can.

Eddie Robinson. Eddie is one of the greatest pro bodybuilders around, and he was kind enough to give us photographs to use in the book.

Finally, I'd like to thank the staff at Perigee Books for believing in a second book and for their time and effort in making it a success.

John Parrillo
Cincinnati, Ohio

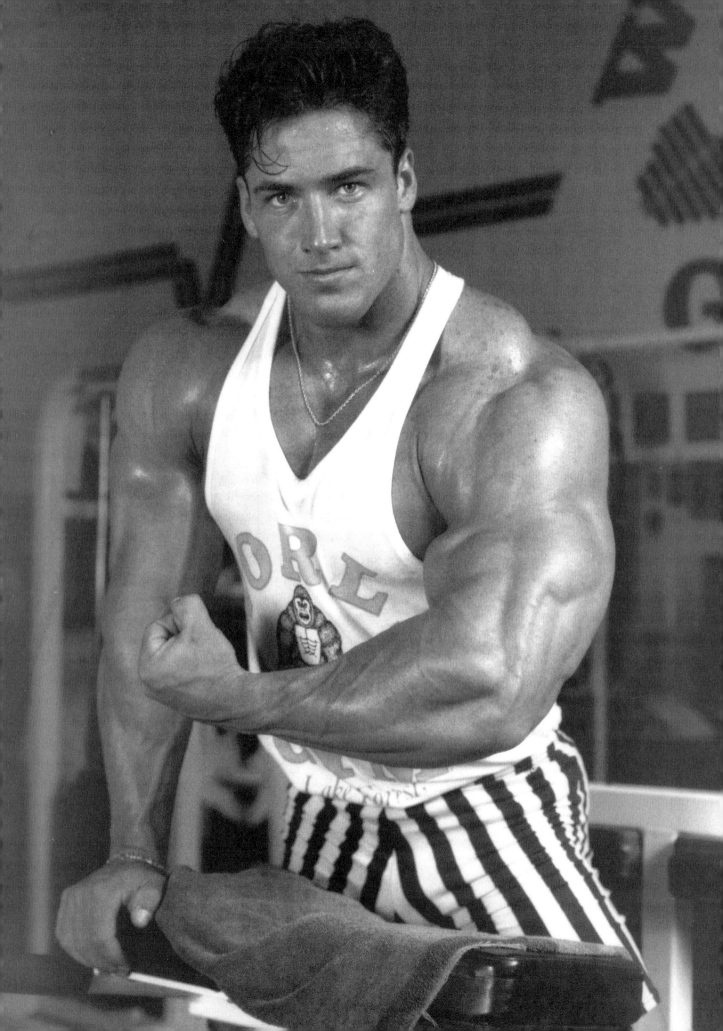

Introduction:
Toward Physique Perfection

Many top professional and amateur bodybuilders have consulted with me over the years, most of them in peak muscular shape. Still, they come to Cincinnati, Ohio, to learn techniques that will further refine their physiques. Most people, upon seeing a top-level bodybuilder, would feel that such athletes are flawless. What kind of help could possibly transform their already near-perfect bodies? And why would they even need help at this pinnacle in their development?

Regardless of your level of training and development, you can still improve your physique, and that applies to anyone. Let's face it, we're all "works in progress."

People who observe my one-on-one work with champions are amazed that I can find flaws in the most highly trained physique. Working with bodybuilders and judging bodybuilding contests for two decades has sharpened my ability to scrutinize physiques. There are some things I can see with my eyes; others, I have to test. Admittedly, I'm looking for flaws, and I'm critical. But bodybuilders don't come to me for praise; they get that from the fans. They come to me because they know I'll give them an honest evaluation of their physiques, and more important, that I'll teach them how to become even better. Through it all, they learn that even a minor change in one variable—nutrition, supplementation, or training—can make a major change in the way they look and perform.

To a degree, bodybuilding is an activity of trial and error. You try umpteen diets, exercises, routines, always searching for that one formula that will magically transform your physique. At long last, that search is over. The techniques explained in this book will produce results for you, as they have for thousands of bodybuilders, in direct proportion to the effort you put forth.

You can achieve your best shape ever. To understand how, let's start by discussing genetics—one of the hurdles on your way to physique perfection, but one that's mostly in your mind.

BREAKING GENETIC BARRIERS

A lot of bodybuilders have a defeatist attitude when it comes to muscles that lag in development. They think lagging muscles are a result of poor genetics, that there's nothing they can do to improve them. Not true! Bodybuilders with so-called lagging muscles are usually not working those muscles hard

Dennis Newman is one of the hottest young stars in bodybuilding. *Photo by Irvin J. Gelb.*

enough—if they're working them at all. They must learn to properly isolate and train those difficult muscle groups for better development.

It has been written that certain elements of genetic makeup such as tendon length and muscle belly cannot be altered. In my experience, however, these can be changed. The only elements that are genetically unalterable are bone length and the insertion point of the muscle (the end attached to the bone that moves).

You can easily change such factors as the shape of your muscle through specialized training and stretching. You can also change your bone structure to some degree, especially the thickness of your sternum and the breadth of your shoulder girdle. It is well known that weight training, along with other weight-bearing exercises, increases bone density by placing mechanical stress on the bones through muscular contraction. As the force from the muscular contraction is increased, more bone mineral (primarily calcium) is taken up by the bones.

The proof of this is found in studies of athletes. One study, for example, found that nationally ranked male tennis players had 35 percent more bone mass in their dominant arms than in their nonplaying arms. In other studies, the greatest bone density has been found in weight lifters, followed in order by throwers, runners, soccer players, and swimmers.[1]

Where body shape is concerned, it's estimated that 20 to 25 percent of your body fat distribution is attributable to genetic factors. You might be born with the tendency toward abdominal or lower body fat, but that doesn't mean you're destined to live with it. You can change fat distribution patterns, and there's no better way to do it than with proper nutrition and specialized training.

Genetic limitations can also be exceeded by increasing nutrient levels in the diet through food and supplementation. When properly nourished, the body starts growing and responding at rates never thought possible.

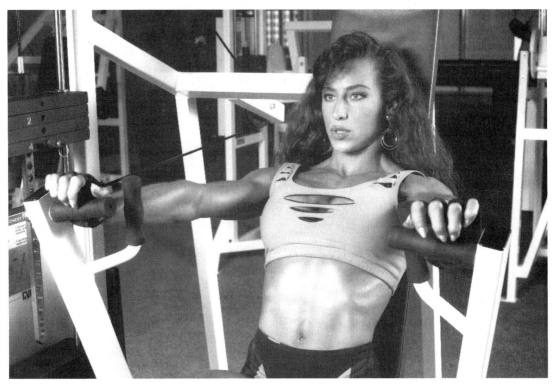

Sherilyn Godreau trains for shape. *Photo by Irvin J. Gelb.*

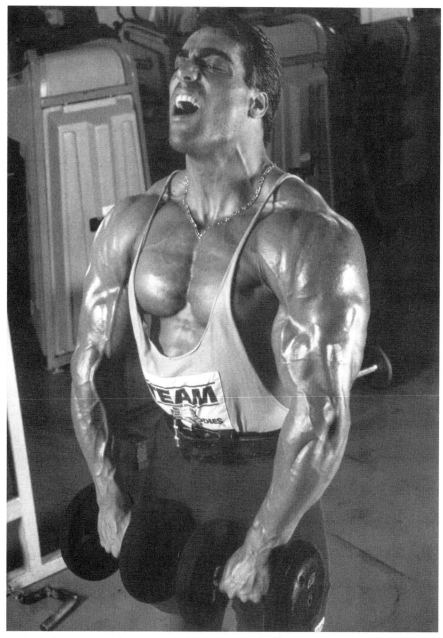

Jimmy Mentis is known as the "Greek God of Bodybuilding." *Photo by Irvin J. Gelb.*

Finally, the mind also plays a vital role in breaking genetic barriers. Athletes work harder trying to break new records after they've beaten earlier ones. It's all in the mind. The only limits in life are those you set mentally. You must believe you can do it, whatever your goal.

ASSESSMENT TECHNIQUES

The first step toward physique perfection is to assess your present development. Assessment gives you a benchmark, a point of reference from which you can measure improvements. When analyzing bodybuilders, I like to assess four interrelated factors: nutrition (including supplementation), muscularity, overall conditioning, and mental acuity.

NUTRITION AND SUPPLEMENTATION

I review a bodybuilder's nutrition first, because it's the foundation for future gains. You have to get your diet right if you want to improve your physique. Proper nutrition involves training your metabolism to burn fat and build muscle more effectively. A diet that achieves this is a high-calorie one (between 2,000 and 10,000 calories a day or more), with five or more meals spread throughout the day and spaced two to three hours apart.

The meals in your diet should include the proper combination of lean proteins (fish, white-meat poultry, and egg whites), starchy carbohydrates (potatoes, yams, rice, legumes, and whole-grain cereals), and fibrous carbohydrates (salad vegetables, broccoli, cauliflower, green beans, etc.). This combination of foods slows your digestion for consistent energy levels and increased endurance throughout the day. It also provides a constant supply of nutrients for muscular growth and repair. Important details on nutrition are covered in Part I.

Supplementation is a component of proper nutrition. Vitamins, minerals and electrolytes, amino acids, medium-chain fatty acids, aspartates, lipotropics, and other supplements increase the nutrient density in cells, activating your body chemistry for growth. I always make sure an athlete is eating the proper foods, however, and not overrelying on supplements for nourishment. Supplements should never take priority over food. But once you're eating correctly, supplements can be added to your diet to maximize the results.

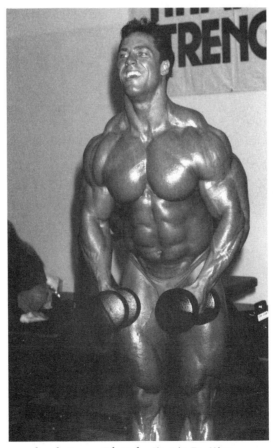

Dennis Newman pumps up backstage. *Photo by Jimmie D. King.*

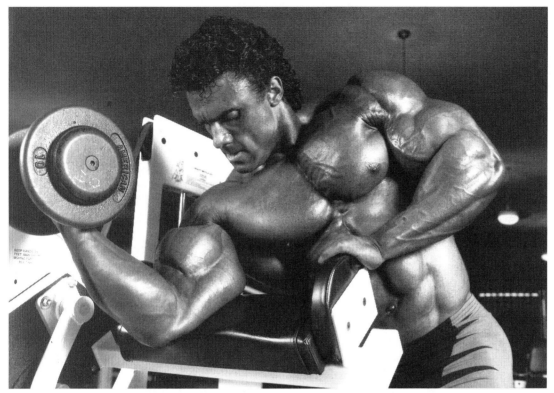

Charles Clairmonte has exceptional biceps mass. *Photo by Irvin J. Gelb.*

MUSCULARITY

"Muscularity" describes the relative development of each muscle—its size, shape, and the degree of body fat present. I can look at a physique and immediately see what areas need work in terms of muscularity. The flaw could be as obvious as poor quadriceps separation. Or it may be barely noticeable, like lagging upper glutes or poor lower lat development. Once I've identified the muscles that need improvement, I review the training techniques that will accomplish the desired result. From that point on, it's up to the bodybuilder to do the work.

If muscularity is obscured by body fat, we discuss nutrition and the strategies that can be taken to reduce body fat. I advise the bodybuilder to:

- Eat fewer starchy carbohydrates. This helps shift the body into a fat-burning mode.
- Increase dietary protein (a nutrient that helps stimulate the metabolism) to promote fat loss while maintaining muscle.
- Gradually increase caloric intake by 200 to 400 calories for a few days to recharge the metabolism for fat-burning.
- Place greater emphasis on heavy weight training to build metabolically active muscle.
- Increase the duration, intensity, and frequency of your aerobics. Doing more aerobic work improves the muscle fibers' ability to oxidize fats for energy, and you get leaner as a result. For more information on aerobics and fat-burning, see section #10.

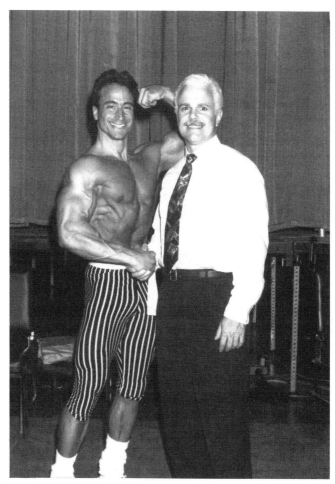

Russ Testo (left) has delighted thousands of bodybuilding fans with his masterful and creative posing. *Photo by Jimmie D. King.*

CONDITIONING

Overall conditioning is critical to the degree of improvement that can be made. That's why I employ an intense assessment process to evaluate certain fitness parameters. To do this, I often put bodybuilders through a multiset routine on a belt squat machine. High-rep, heavy-poundage sets are used, and these let me evaluate the following:

Strength. I load the bodybuilder up with weight, usually beginning at 100 pounds. Each set, I increase the poundages to see how much weight can be handled. During the workout, I observe a strength factor known as the "Golgi tendon reflex (GTR) threshold." This is a physiological response to weight-bearing stress placed on the tendons as a result of muscular contractions.

Between the muscle and the tendons, there is a group of sensory receptors called Golgi tendon organs. During strenuous, high-intensity workouts, Golgi tendon organs fire when the tendon is stretched too far, shutting the muscle down to prevent injury.

You might have felt this response during very heavy training. At a certain point, your muscles shake and eventually give out on an exercise. In addition to being fatigued, they have been purposely switched off by your Golgi tendon organs as a protective measure.

The strength or weakness of your tendons can be gauged by the point at which the Golgi tendon organs kick in. If your muscles shut down quickly while you're using fairly light poundages, then you have a low GTR threshold. Obviously, this can be a limiting factor in training, because it reduces the ability to continue muscular contractions and to handle heavy weights.

As a bodybuilder, one of your goals should be to increase your GTR threshold so that you can increase your strength and perform heavier, more intense workouts. This can be accomplished by utilizing power techniques such as heavy reps, forced reps, singles, triples, and negatives. For additional information on how to build strength, see section #43.

General Cardiovascular Conditioning. Descriptive of the capacity to use oxygen, general cardiovascular conditioning relates directly to metabolic efficiency. Proper conditioning allows optimal combination of oxygen with nutrients for the production of energy. As a result, food calories are used more efficiently and are less likely to be stored as body fat.

If your breathing gives out too soon while you're performing high-rep sets and you can't take in enough oxygen to continue, then your general cardiovascular conditioning needs some rehauling. More aerobics in the overall training program will correct this response. Section #10 includes additional information about general cardiovascular conditioning.

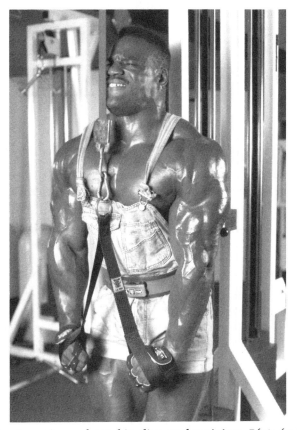

Massive Chris Cormier is serious about his diet and training. *Photo by Irvin J. Gelb.*

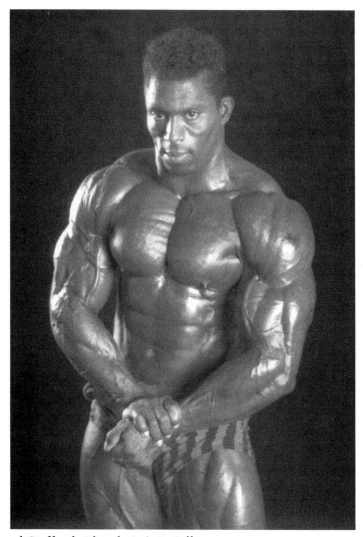

Bodybuilder Darryl Stafford. *Photo by Irvin J. Gelb.*

Specific Cardiovascular Conditioning. Next, I evaluate specific cardiovascular conditioning—the ability of a single muscle group (in this case the legs) to clear out waste products from the muscles as you train them. The faster waste products leave the muscle, the easier it is to continue muscular contractions.

By the last set of the belt squat, I can gauge the level of specific cardiovascular conditioning. The number of reps in this set is high—between 40 and 100. Spotters are rotated in at 20-rep intervals to keep the bodybuilder going. Sometimes a bodybuilder's legs start burning so early in the workout that he quits. This is a symptom of poor specific cardiovascular conditioning. Waste products like lactic acid, which produce the burn, are not being cleared from the muscles efficiently.

If your muscles burn too early in a set, you need to incorporate more high-rep training into your routines to build specific cardiovascular conditioning. Guidelines on how to improve specific cardiovascular conditioning are covered in section #11.

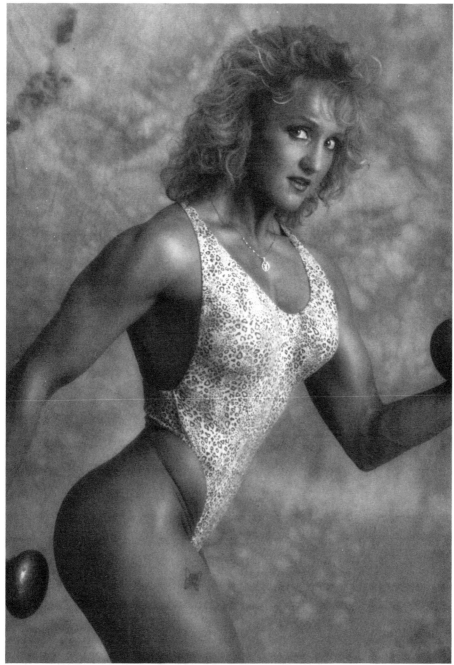

Tony Dee is a favorite in West Coast bodybuilding circles. *Photo by Paul B. Goode.*

Flexibility. As part of the assessment, I stretch the bodybuilder to determine the flexibility or tightness of the fascia, the connective tissue that envelops the muscles. The more flexible it is, the more room there is under the fascial sheath for muscular growth. A bodybuilder can stretch the fascial tissue by using a special technique I developed called "fascial stretching." It involves intense stretching between sets when the muscle is fully pumped. By opening up the area between the fascia and the muscle it surrounds, fascial stretching dramatically enhances muscular growth, size, separation, and strength. Several key fascial stretching exercises are reviewed in section #14.

MENTAL ACUITY

Throughout the assessment, I analyze the bodybuilder's mental acuity—the concentration applied to the workout and the belief in one's own physical capacity. Bodybuilders who want to stop before they have totally fatigued themselves should work to increase their mental acuity. Mental acuity underpins everything in training, so stay focused and believe that you can go further and harder than ever before. Mental acuity and motivational recommendations are explained in section #50.

By observing someone's performance during a session like this, I can make precise recommendations on points that need improvement. It is then up to the bodybuilder to work on these weak points.

You can assess your own conditioning in the same way. Working with a partner, put yourself through a high-rep leg routine on a belt squat machine, conventional squat, or other leg machine. Push yourself to the max. See what you can tolerate, physically and mentally.

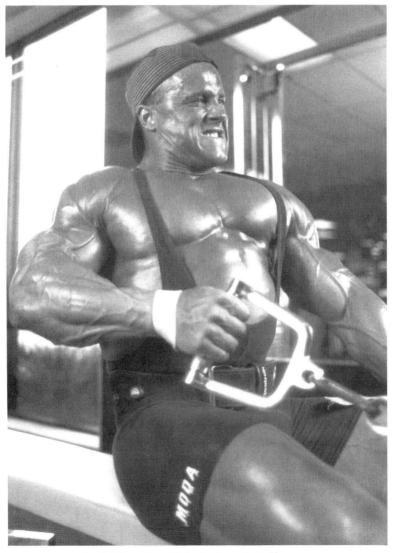

Mental acuity is a key part of intensity. *Photo by Irvin J. Gelb.*

As you strive for new levels of intensity and performance, make sure you're taking in enough nutrients from your diet and supplements to support the intensity of your training. The harder you train, the more nutrients you'll require. As you increase your nutrients, you'll experience greater energy and endurance in the gym.

Now let's take a look at the 50 techniques and strategies you can use to build a near-perfect physique.

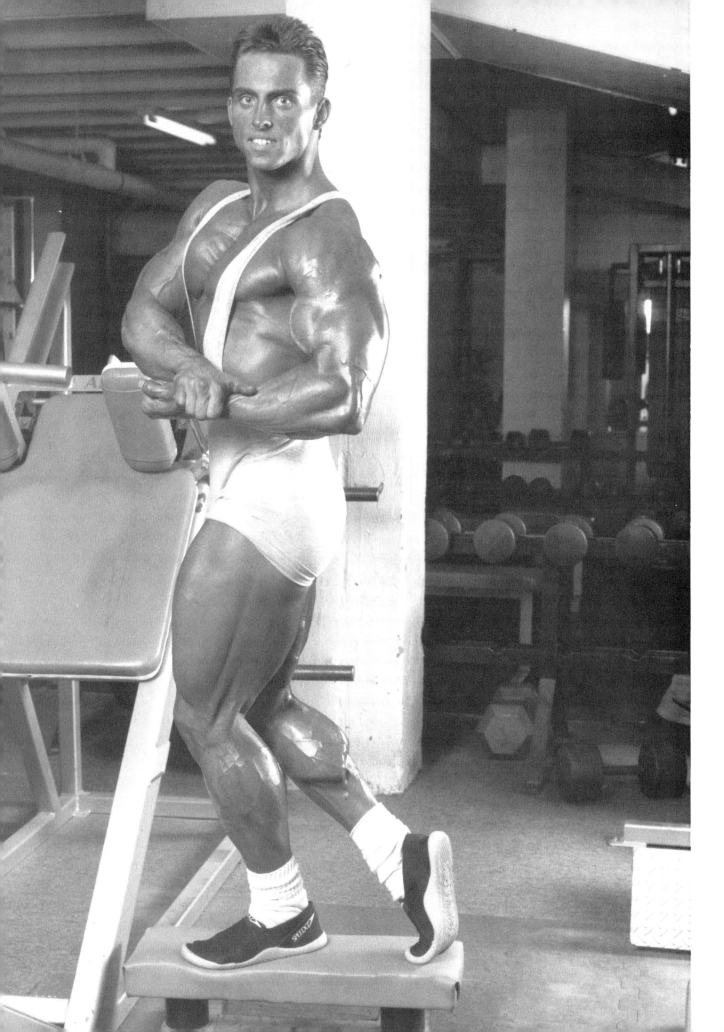

PART
I
NUTRITION
SECRETS

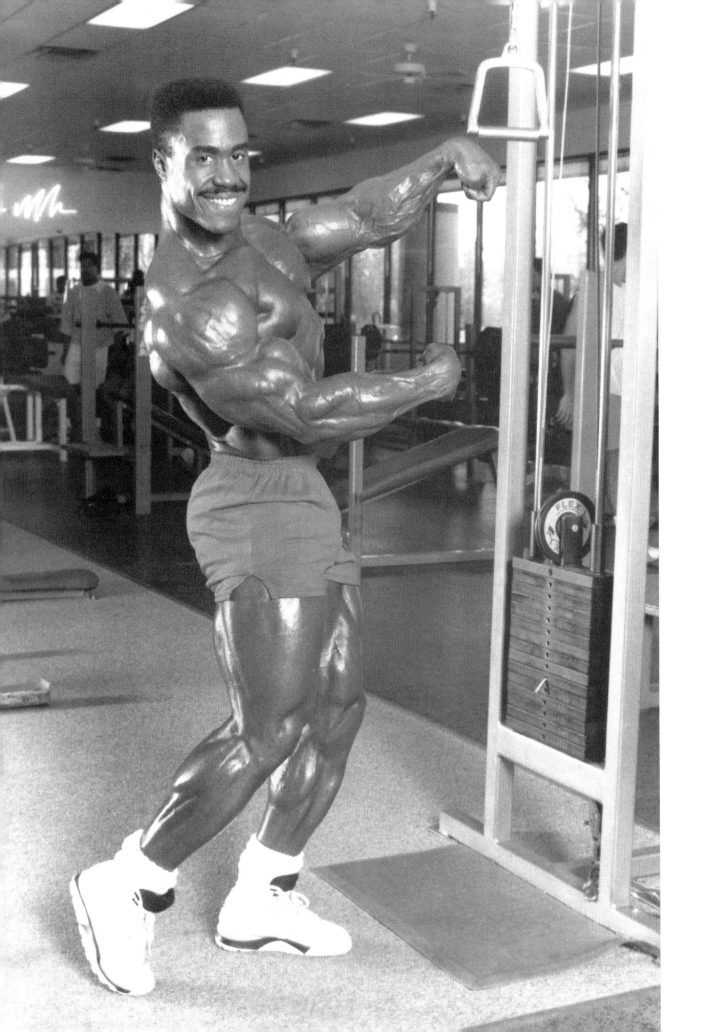

1 THE POWER OF FOOD

Beware of the latest nutrition fad hyping a "miracle" supplement—any product promising to magically transform your body so that it's leaner and more muscular. There's no such thing. But there is a substance you need for growth—food. To get the results you want from nutrition, food will always work much more effectively than "miracle" supplements or meal replacement diets. I call food the "perfect supplement."

Food provides something that supplements or meal replacement diets do not: the raw materials your body needs for growth and for the stimulation of chemical processes involved in the breakdown, absorption, and assimilation of nutrients. The digestive process, for example, requires "real" food—complete with its balance of nutrients and fiber—to do the job for which it was designed. The presence of food, acids, and digestive enzymes in the duodenum (the first section of the small intestine) and the jejunum (the second section of the small intestine) stimulates the production of hormones required for the absorption of nutrients. Without food, these processes are interrupted, and the proper assimilation of nutrients is impaired. Your body's cells don't get everything they need.

In my work with the best bodybuilders and athletes in the world, I've identified which foods yield the best results in terms of physique and performance. Lean protein, for example, supplies nutrients called "amino acids," which are required for every metabolic process. Athletes have higher requirements for protein than the average person. Without enough protein, you cannot build muscle, repair its breakdown after training, or drive your metabolism. Starchy and fibrous carbohydrates supply energy and are stored as glycogen in the muscles and liver.

You need certain fats called "essential fatty acids" (EFAs), which must be supplied by the diet. EFAs regulate many biological functions, including the manufacture of connective tissue, cellular walls, and hormones. You can get EFAs from safflower oil, flaxseed oil, linseed oil, and sunflower seed oil, among others.

All the foods I recommend have a "high nutrient density." This describes the ratio of nutrients in a food to the energy it supplies. Natural starchy foods like potatoes, yams, brown rice, and whole grains are packed with carbohydrates, protein, vitamins, and minerals. Fibrous vegetables are rich in vitamins, minerals, water, fiber, and carbohydrates. And lean proteins are high not only in protein but in vitamins and minerals. In short, high-nutrient-density foods pack a lot of nutritional wallop, and that's why you should eat them.

Try to stay away from low-nutrient-density foods: processed foods, sweets, soft drinks, alcoholic beverages, and high-fat foods. Low-nutrient-density foods are easily converted to body fat or, as in the case of alcohol, can interfere with the body's ability to metabolize fat.

Foods containing simple sugars are excluded from my nutrition program be-

Mike Ashley's devotion to natural bodybuilding has propelled him to success in the sport. *Photo by Irvin J. Gelb.*

cause they also convert easily to body fat. These foods include fruit and fruit juices, which contain the simple sugar fructose, and dairy products, which contain the simple sugar lactose.

You can increase the nutrient density of your nutrition by adding in supplements—but only after you're eating properly. By taking supplements, you force your digestive system to process more nutrients. This allows the nutrient levels in your body to be increased at the cellular level—beyond what can be achieved by eating food alone—which, along with a gradual increase of calories, helps your body grow. Supplements are quality nutrients that work in conjunction with food to help your body build its metabolism and recovery mechanisms.

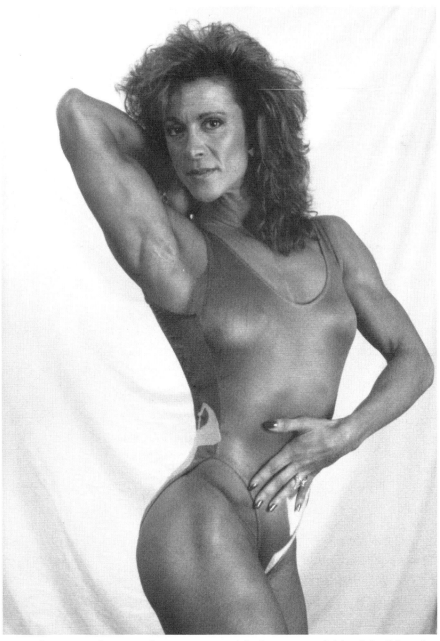

Consistency and intensity have made pro Janet Tech the successful bodybuilder she is today. *Photo by Jimmie D. King.*

Other important dietary issues are involved as well. Foods such as legumes and other starchy carbohydrates contain special complex sugars called "oligosaccharides." These sugars exert a healthful effect on the growth of beneficial bacteria in the gastrointestinal (GI) tract. One family of these bacteria is called "bifidobacterium." Because of the oligosaccharides' effect on this type of bacteria, the sugars have been called "bifidus factors." When bifidobacteria and other helpful bacteria are present in the GI tract, they prevent dangerous and sometimes deadly bacteria such as salmonella and E. *coli* from colonizing.

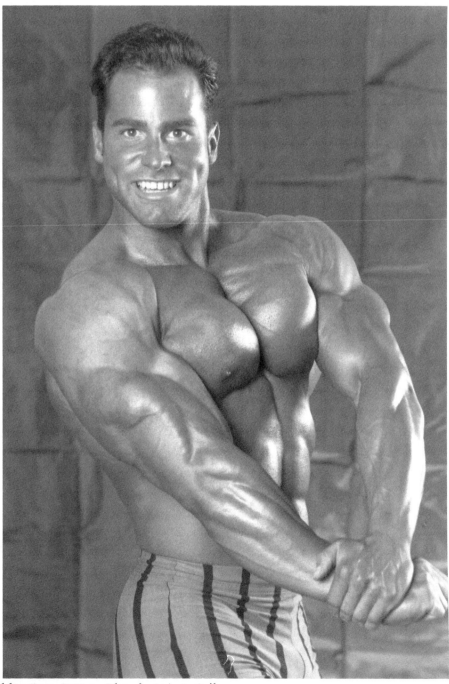

Bodybuilder Tom Pattyn. *Photo by Irvin J. Gelb.*

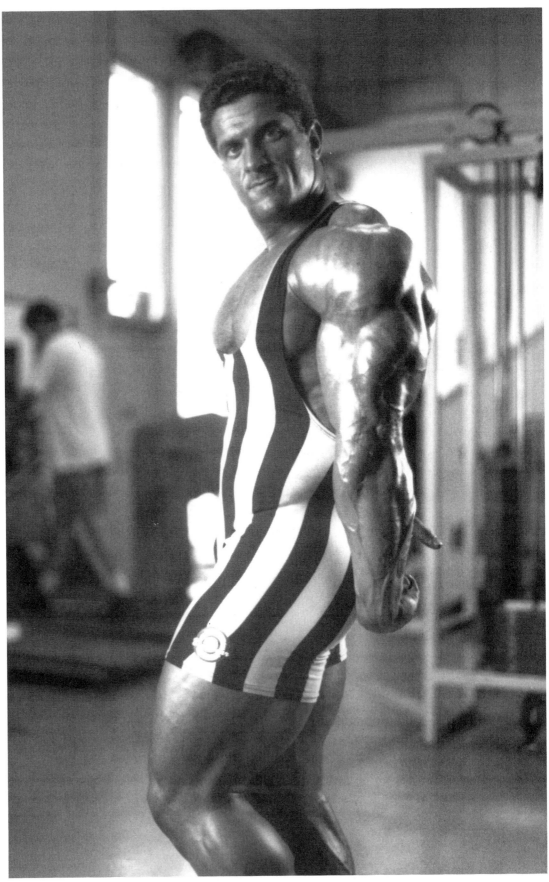

Joe Spinello displays balanced, full triceps development. *Photo by Irvin J. Gelb.*

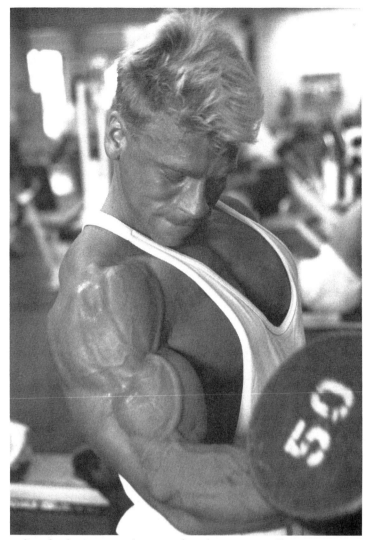

A nutrient-dense diet fuels your workouts. *Photo by Irvin J. Gelb.*

Human milk is another food that contains oligosaccharides. It's well known that breast-fed infants quickly develop a protective population of bifidobacteria. Oligosaccharides have also been shown to protect cells from the invasion of the bacteria responsible for certain types of pneumonia, influenza, and other serious respiratory tract infections.

The bacterial population of the GI tract obviously plays an important role in nutrition and health. Scientists are now exploring the use of oligosaccharides in the treatment of digestive disorders, elevated blood fats, and other health problems. The ability of oligosaccharides to promote healthy bacterial growth underlines the importance of food as the source for these protective factors. In other words, you cannot obtain such factors from supplements.

Food is the cornerstone of nutrition. If you don't eat the proper foods—lean proteins, starchy carbohydrates, and fibrous carbohydrates—nothing else matters. No supplement can ever provide all the benefits that food supplies. We were built to process food—proteins, carbohydrates, and fats.

If you want to make the best possible progress with your physique, I suggest that you start with the basics. And that means food.

2 NUTRIENT PARTITIONING: THE ULTIMATE BODYBUILDING DIET

To a degree, you have a great deal of control over whether the food you eat is turned into body fat or muscle. The assignment of food to either fat stores or muscle stores is called "nutrient partitioning," and it's the secret behind getting lean and staying muscular.

To understand how nutrient partitioning works, it's helpful to think of the body as being divided into a fat compartment and a lean compartment. Food goes to either of these compartments or is burned for energy.

One of the factors that has a significant effect on nutrient partitioning is your endocrine system. It's involved in such processes as metabolism, energy production, and growth. The endocrine system consists of several organs in the body, including the pituitary gland, the thyroid gland, the parathyroid gland, the pancreas, the testes or ovaries, and the kidneys. This specialized system is like a chemical "messenger service" in the body: It transmits messages in the form of hormones, carried by the blood to specific targets (organs, tissues, or cells) in the body. The messages sent are things like "build muscle proteins," "store fat," "burn fat," or "store carbohydrates."

Once these messages are received by the targets, the commands are carried out by enzymes, special proteins that control chemical reactions inside cells. Through these reactions, enzymes can make or break down proteins or fat.

Two of the most important hormones involved in muscle growth and fat loss are insulin and glucagon, both produced in the pancreas. They regulate carbohydrate metabolism and fat metabolism by exerting control over the enzymes that carry out these processes.

When blood sugar (glucose) levels rise—usually after carbohydrates are eaten—insulin is released. It transports glucose into cells where it is burned for energy or stored as glycogen. If carbohydrates are released into the bloodstream too fast, an overproduction of insulin occurs. Consequently, some of the carbohydrates are deposited as fat—instead of being stored as glycogen. Simple sugars and refined carbohydrates are rapid-release foods that trigger too much insulin. This channels calories to the fat compartment of the body—not the avenue of nutrient partitioning you want.

Interestingly, insulin is involved in muscular growth because it transports certain amino acids into muscle cells. To make this happen, you need carbohydrates. The key, however, is eating the right kinds of carbs, in the right amounts.

Glucagon opposes the effect of insulin. When blood sugar is low, glucagon is released, typically several hours after a meal is eaten. Glucagon then activates the conversion of glycogen to glucose in the liver in response to low blood sugar levels. It also signals the body to start burning fat for energy, because the body is running low on carbohydrates, its preferred fuel source.

The ratio of insulin to glycogen in your body largely determines whether you will gain fat or lose it. You can control this ratio naturally by adjusting the protein and carbohydrate proportions in your diet and combining foods in the proper manner. Here's how you can partition your food more effectively, so it can be used to burn fat and build muscle:

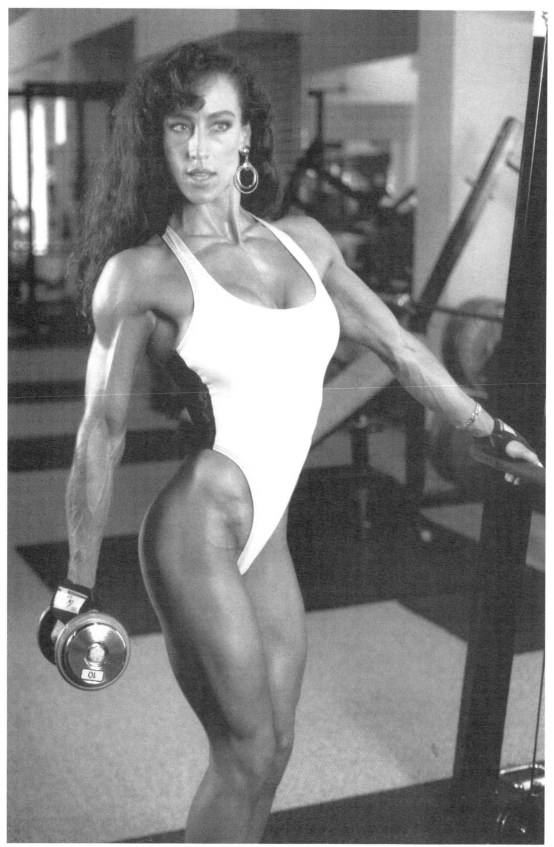

Sherilyn Godreau is one of the most popular fitness stars around. *Photo by Irvin J. Gelb.*

1. When trying to gain muscular weight, you want a higher ratio of insulin, so you would increase your carbohydrate intake, perhaps as high as 400 to 500 grams or more a day. A carbohydrate supplement formulated with the complex carbohydrate maltodextrin is a good way to increase carbohydrate consumption. At the same time, be sure to meet your lean-protein requirements by eating between 1.25 and 1.5 grams of protein per pound of body weight. At least 1 gram should come from chicken, fish, turkey, or egg whites, with at least another .25 or .5 gram of additional protein per pound of body weight from vegetable sources, which contain some protein as well.

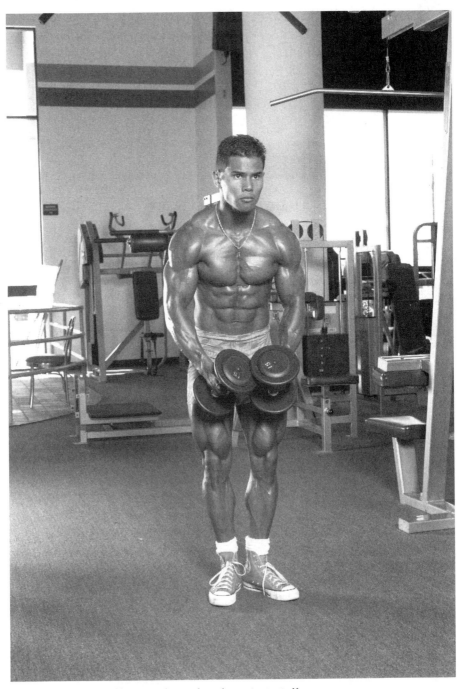

Al Escobar, Jr., is lean and muscular. *Photo by Irvin J. Gelb.*

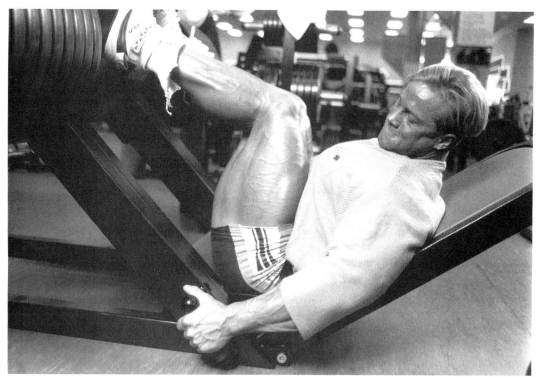

Proper nutrition fuels you for heavy, intense training. *Photo by Irvin J. Gelb.*

2. To lose body fat, decrease insulin and increase glucagon by eating slightly less carbohydrate and more protein. A good rule of thumb is to adjust your carbohydrate-to-protein ratio to between 1 to 1 and 1.5 to 1. One problem with reducing carbohydrate intake is the potential decline in energy levels. To compensate, try supplementing your diet with medium-chain triglyceride oil (better known as "MCT oil" or "MCFA oil"). This is a special type of lipid that provides quality calories and, unlike conventional dietary fats, is not likely to be stored as body fat.

3. Don't take nutrient partitioning to extremes by going on a "zero carb" diet in an attempt to burn more body fat. Under extremely low-carb conditions, muscular growth is impossible. There's not enough insulin available to transport amino acids into muscle cells. Furthermore, the body begins to break down its own proteins into amino acids for conversion into glucose, needed by the brain for fuel.

4. Rate of digestion is important. Your meals (five, six, or more a day) should include the proper combination of lean proteins, starchy carbohydrates, and fibrous carbohydrates. This combination of foods slows your digestion to keep carbohydrates from being released into the bloodstream too fast, thus preventing an overproduction of insulin.

3 ACHIEVING PERMANENT FAT LOSS

One of the biggest mysteries in modern medicine today is how to successfully treat people who are overweight. We used to think the culprit behind this condition was overeating. People ate too much, so they got fat. Given that assumption, dieters were told to restrict calories to lose weight. In theory, the approach made sense—except for one thing. Medical research now shows that for the most part there's no correlation between food intake and being overweight. In other words, most overweight people don't eat any more than people of average weight do.

The cut-calorie approach to weight loss has begun to fall apart for another reason: Nearly 95 percent of those who go on low-calorie diets regain their lost weight, plus some, within five years. Not a resounding endorsement for low-calorie dieting.

Why do people put weight back on so readily? There are several possible answers. To begin with, 25 to 50 percent of body weight lost by cutting calories is muscle. Since muscle is the body's most metabolically active tissue, losing so much of it slows the metabolism down.

Moreover, cutting calories tricks your body into thinking it's starving. This perceived famine speeds up the activity of a special enzyme that primes your body to store fat. Once you go off your diet and start eating again, the food is converted more easily to fat. In fact, fat stores stand first in line to be replaced after a period of dieting. You return to your original body weight or reach a higher weight, this time with even more body fat than before.

Restricting calories affects this relapse in other ways, too. Less food energy is given off as body heat: Instead, it's turned into weight. Low-calorie diets also suppress the activity of certain thyroid hormones, further slowing down the metabolism.

The type of food you eat also influences your tendency to put on body fat. Although excess calories from any food can be stored as body fat, some foods are converted more readily than others. Dietary fat is the easiest fat to store because it has the same chemical structure as body fat. The more fat you eat, the more fat you'll wear.

By contrast, protein and carbohydrate have to be chemically converted to fat before they can be stored as fat. This conversion process uses up some of the calories in the protein and carbohydrate food, reducing the tendency of these foods to be deposited as fat.

In addition, carbohydrates are burned for energy more efficiently by the body than dietary fat is. In fact, most active people can eat as much as 500 grams of carbohydrate a day without gaining fat. Eating foods that are easily burned and avoiding foods that are easily stored will help you knock off fat pounds.

Given all these factors, I'd say the decks are pretty well stacked against low-calorie dieting. So what do you do? Whether you're a competitive bodybuilder trying to get down to 4 percent body fat or someone just trying to get in better shape, you *can* achieve permanent fat loss. Here's how:

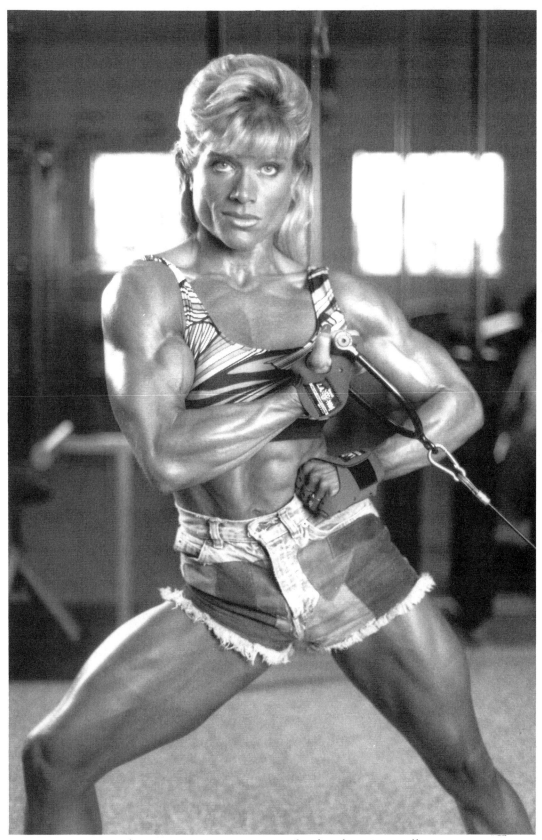

Drorit Kernes's muscular separation is exceptional. *Photo by Irvin J. Gelb.*

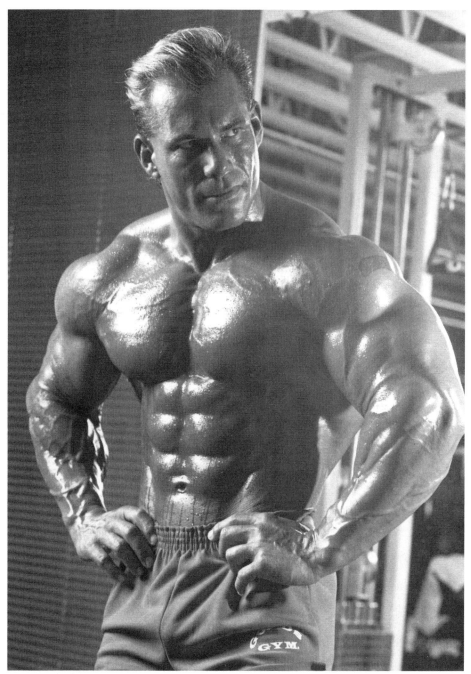

Bodybuilder Rick Stephenson. *Photo by Ralph DeHaan.*

1. Clearly, you can't stay lean by cutting calories. That's why I recommend a program of gradually increasing calories to build the metabolism for faster fat-burning. Your goal should be to lose body fat slowly—at the rate of one pound a week. One pound of body fat contains 3,500 calories. To lose that pound, you need a calorie deficit of 500 a day. Get that deficit through exercise, from both weight training and aerobics. One hour a day of intense aerobic activity will burn 500 calories. Be sure to monitor your body composition (percentages of lean mass and body fat) to make sure that you're not losing muscle. If you are, you'll need to further increase your calories, especially since the more aerobics you do, the more nutrients you'll require. An accurate way to check your body composition is by using my BodyStat Charting System in the Appendix.

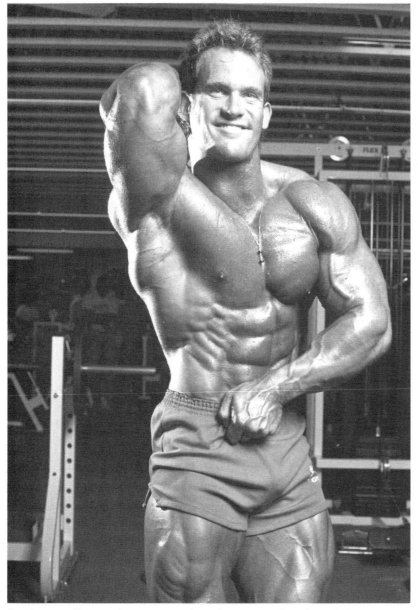

Tight abs show up well on a lean, muscular physique. *Photo by Ralph DeHaan.*

2. Increase the ratio of complex carbohydrates to fat in your diet. Remember, carbs are burned more efficiently than fat is. If you need to lose body fat, limit your fat intake to about 5 percent of your total food consumption.

3. Avoid simple sugars, which are more readily converted to body fat. (For an explanation of how this occurs, see section #4.) Stick to starchy and fibrous carbohydrates.

4. Plan a protein-to-carbohydrate ratio that will result in an insulin/glucagon ratio compatible with fat loss. Remember, insulin promotes fat storage while glucagon increases the use of fat for energy. A good rule of thumb is to plan a diet consisting of 30 percent lean protein, 65 percent complex carbohydrates, and 5 percent fat. (See section #2 on nutrient partitioning.)

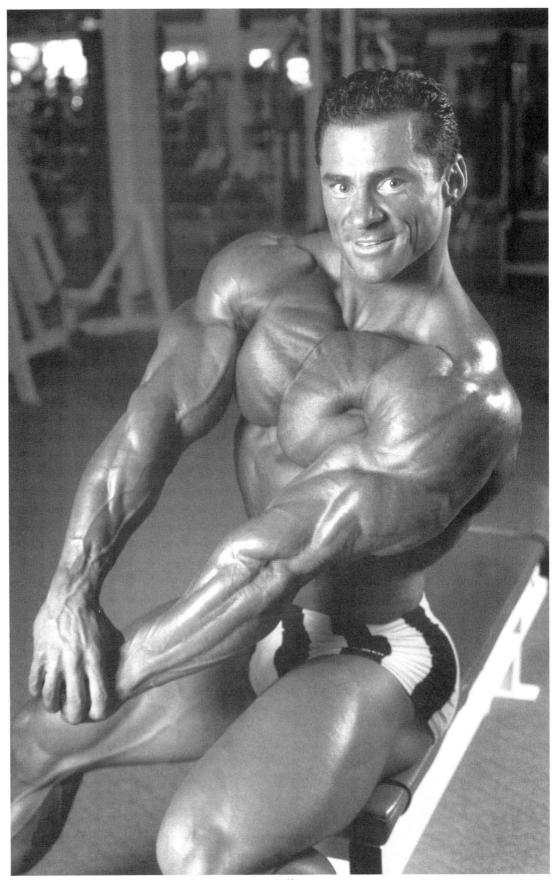

Bodybuilder James Harrison. *Photo by Irvin J. Gelb.*

4 THE TRUTH ABOUT FRUCTOSE

I'm frequently asked to explain why fruits and fruit juices are not included in my nutrition program. The answer has to do with a little-understood simple sugar found in fruit: fructose.

Fructose came into favor years ago because of its stabilizing effect on blood sugar. Unlike other simple sugars, it triggers neither a surge of insulin nor a corresponding drop in blood sugar an hour or so after eating it. That's the good news. But there's more to the fructose story.

After you work out, your body moves from an energy-using mode (catabolism) to an energy storage and rebuilding mode (anabolism). During the transition, dietary carbohydrate is broken down into glucose and fructose to be used for "glycogenesis," the manufacture of glycogen to restock the muscles and liver.

Fructose is used primarily to restore liver glycogen; it's really not a good resupplier of muscle glycogen. Glucose, on the other hand, bypasses the liver and is carried by the bloodstream straight to the muscles you just worked, where the glycogen-making process begins. Any muscle emptied of glycogen by exercise is first on the list to get its quota of glucose.

Clearly, one of the keys to effectively restoring glycogen is the type of carbohydrate you eat. Natural, starchy carbohydrates such as potatoes, yams, whole grains, corn, and legumes do a better job at this than simple sugars do. Research has shown that a diet high in starchy carbohydrates can restock more glycogen in the muscles forty-eight hours after exercise than simple sugars can.[1]

If you eat simple sugars like fructose, you're not going to be able to store as much glycogen had you consumed natural, starchy carbohydrates. What implications does this have for you as an athlete or bodybuilder?

First, you won't be able to train as hard or as long during your next workout, because you haven't stored as much glycogen. Nor will you be able to recover from your workouts as efficiently. Moreover, the simple sugars are likely to spill over into fat stores, with just a fraction converted to glycogen. By contrast, eating ample amounts of starchy carbohydrates will extend your endurance and effectively resupply your muscles with glycogen for better recovery. You'll stay leaner, too, since starchy carbs are fully utilized for energy production and glycogen synthesis.

Second, you'll notice less of a "pump" while working out, also because of low glycogen stores in the muscle. The "pump" describes an exercised muscle heavily engorged with blood. If you can't get a good pump, it's difficult to get the full benefits of "fascial stretching," my system of stretching between exercise sets. Fascial stretching stretches the fascia tissue surrounding the muscle so that it has more room to grow. The best time to stretch is when the muscle is fully pumped, because the pump helps stretch the fascia, too. With low glycogen levels in the muscle, you can't stretch to the maximum. This limits your growth potential. (For more information on fascial stretching, see section #14.)

Third, fructose is easily converted to body fat. Because of fructose's molecular structure, the liver readily converts it into a long-chain triglyceride (a fat).

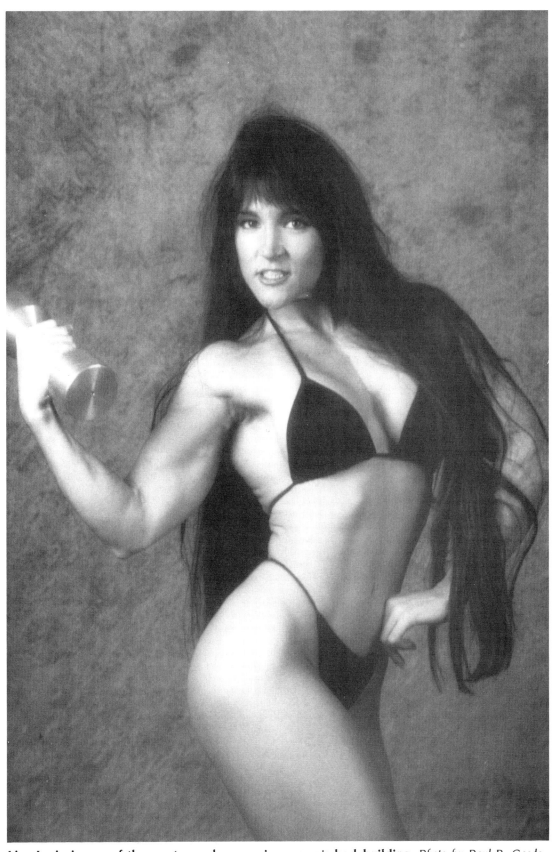

Lisa Lorio is one of the most popular pros in women's bodybuilding. *Photo by Paul B. Goode.*

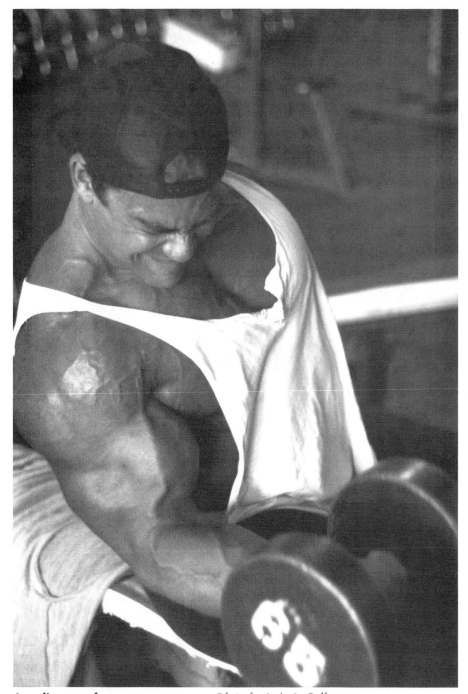

Joe De Angelis goes for more arm mass. *Photo by Irvin J. Gelb.*

Therefore, a majority of the fruit you eat can ultimately end up as body fat on your physique. You'll notice an incredible difference when you eliminate fruits and juices from your diet.

That's not to say fruit isn't healthful. It's high in vitamins, minerals, and fiber—but so are natural, complex carbohydrates. If you want to get leaner and more muscular—and build your recuperative powers by restocking glycogen more efficiently—avoid fruit. Choose starchy and fibrous carbohydrates instead.

5 PROTEIN AND MUSCULAR HARDNESS

Large, well-shaped muscles mean little without a quality called "muscular hardness"—a tight, rock-solid firmness that can't be obtained by training but through proper nutrition. Here's a case in point:

Recently, I worked with a bodybuilder who prepared for a national contest by performing intense, two-hour workouts in the gym, along with two hours of daily aerobics. He weighed 240 pounds, with massive muscles from head to toe.

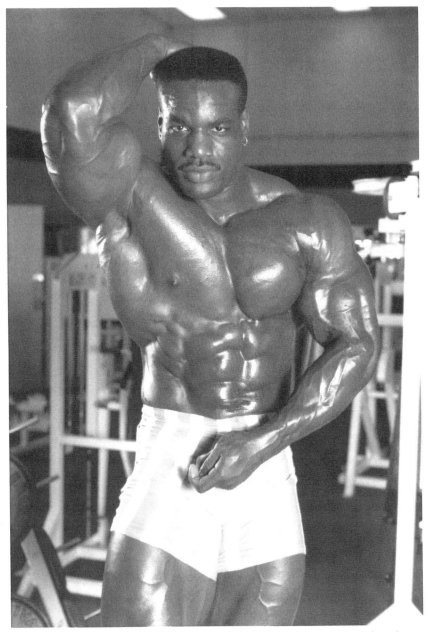

Muscular hardness can be achieved by consuming adequate protein. *Photo by Irvin J. Gelb.*

Despite his development, his muscles were soft, and no amount of training seemed to help. We made just one change—to his diet—and that change made all the difference in the world. We increased his protein intake from 350 grams a day to 600 grams a day, and he hardened up in a matter of days. His physique took on a totally new, more dramatic look. As I've pointed out, a minor change can make a major difference.

Protein, because of its role in supplying amino acids for growth and repair, is the key to muscular hardness. Which brings up a key question: How much protein do bodybuilders actually need?

The National Research Council sets the recommended daily allowance (RDA) at .8 grams per kilogram of body weight—the equivalent of .36 grams per pound. Based on the RDA, a 200-pound bodybuilder would require a mere 72

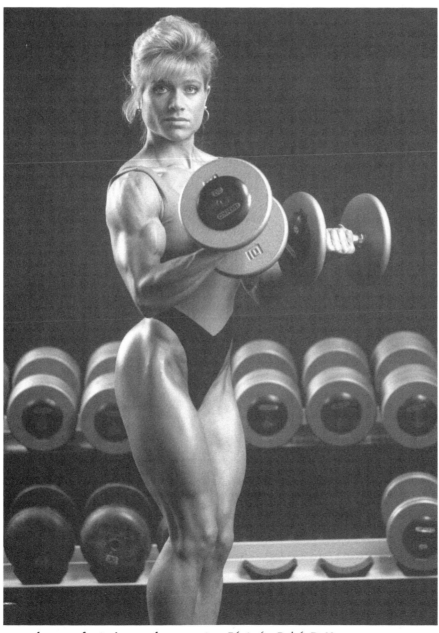

Drorit Kernes has perfect size and symmetry. *Photo by Ralph DeHaan.*

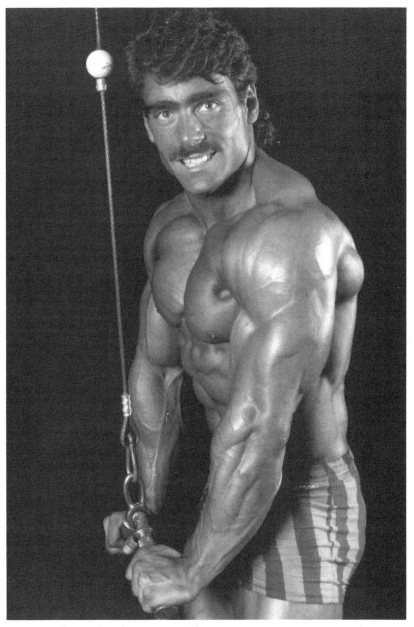

Bodybuilder Rob Mello. *Photo by Irvin J. Gelb.*

grams of protein a day—the equivalent of three small chicken breasts. Unfortunately, the RDA was established with average, sedentary people in mind.

Other methods, based on nitrogen balance studies, are now being used to determine the protein requirements for athletes. Nitrogen balance means that the body is rebuilding at the same rate of breakdown. If tissue breakdown is faster than tissue buildup, you're losing more nitrogen than you get from food. This state is called "negative nitrogen balance," and it's often induced by restrictive dieting. If less nitrogen is eliminated than is taken in, you're in a "positive nitrogen balance," indicating the growth of new muscle tissue. Nitrogen balance studies show that the protein requirement for athletes may be 23 to 178 percent greater than for the average population.

Recent research indicates that weight-training athletes need greater amounts of protein. In one study, for example, ten weight lifters trained intensely and consumed .9 grams of protein per pound of body weight a day. Four of these athletes were found to be in negative nitrogen balance.[1]

In another study, weight lifters who increased their protein intake from 1.0 to 1.6 grams per pound of body weight a day were able to increase both strength and lean mass. Two other studies, both involving bodybuilders, found that eating 1.2 grams of protein per pound of body weight produced greater nitrogen retention than consuming .45 grams per pound of body weight a day.[2]

Serious bodybuilders train aerobically as well, and this places some additional demands on the protein needs of the body. Prolonged aerobic exercise, for example, can burn amino acids after the body uses up its stored carbohydrate (glycogen), thus elevating protein requirements.

Aerobic training in a protein-deficient state can lead to a condition called "sports anemia," in which red blood cells and iron levels are reduced. One explanation for this is that aerobic training appears to increase myoglobin, an oxygen-carrying protein in the muscles. The formation of myoglobin requires protein and heme iron (this is iron that is bound to heme, the special pigment in red blood cells). If protein is in short supply, red blood cells are destroyed to obtain the necessary protein and iron to make myoglobin.

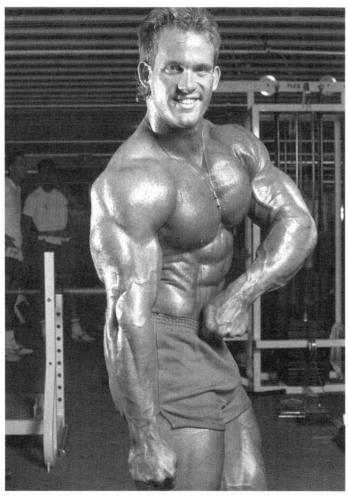

Bodybuilder John DePolo. *Photo by Ralph DeHaan.*

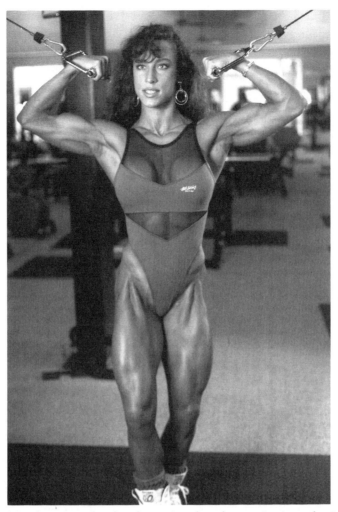

Sherilyn Godreau has the muscular hardness it takes for a winning physique. *Photo by Irvin J. Gelb.*

In addition, muscle fibers are damaged during training and must be repaired following the exercise period. If your protein intake is low, the body draws on red blood cells and blood proteins as a source of protein for muscular repair. When this happens, little protein is left to rebuild red blood cells at the normal rate, and sports anemia can be the result.

Clearly, bodybuilders and other athletes must include ample protein in their diets to promote muscular fitness. Individual protein needs vary and depend on a number of factors, including a bodybuilder's training intensity and level of conditioning. I've seen many bodybuilders improve their physiques by increasing their protein intake up to 2.5 grams per pound of body weight a day— nearly seven times the RDA.

Without an adequate intake of protein, you won't be able to build or repair muscle. But if you consume too much, the excess could be stored as fat. Based on my experience, hard-training bodybuilders can achieve excellent results— including muscular hardness—by consuming 1.25 to 1.5 grams of protein per pound of body weight a day. One gram per pound of body weight should come from lean-protein sources such as white-meat poultry, fish, and egg whites; the other .25 to .5 gram per pound of body weight can come from all your other foods, particularly high-protein vegetables like beans, corn, and legumes.

6 THE ENERGY TO TRAIN ALL OUT

Partway into your workout, have you ever felt your energy levels waning? If so, it's time to reexamine your nutrition. To maintain an intense level of training, including aerobics and weight training, you must fuel your body with ample calories from the right foods: lean proteins, starchy carbohydrates, and fibrous carbohydrates, eaten in combination five, six, or more times a day. Additionally, certain supplements play a key role when added to proper nutrition. These are covered in the next section. What follows are some important nutritional guidelines that will help you train longer and harder, without feeling sapped while in the gym.

Protein. If you include a lot of aerobics in your training program, you can learn from the experience of endurance athletes, who actually have even higher protein requirements than most strength athletes. The reason is that amino acids (the building blocks of protein) are used as fuel during endurance training. As you plan your daily diet, make sure you're taking in my recommended levels of protein.

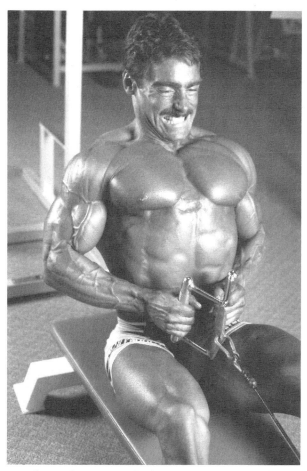

Stamina comes from quality calories—and plenty of them. *Photo by Irvin J. Gelb.*

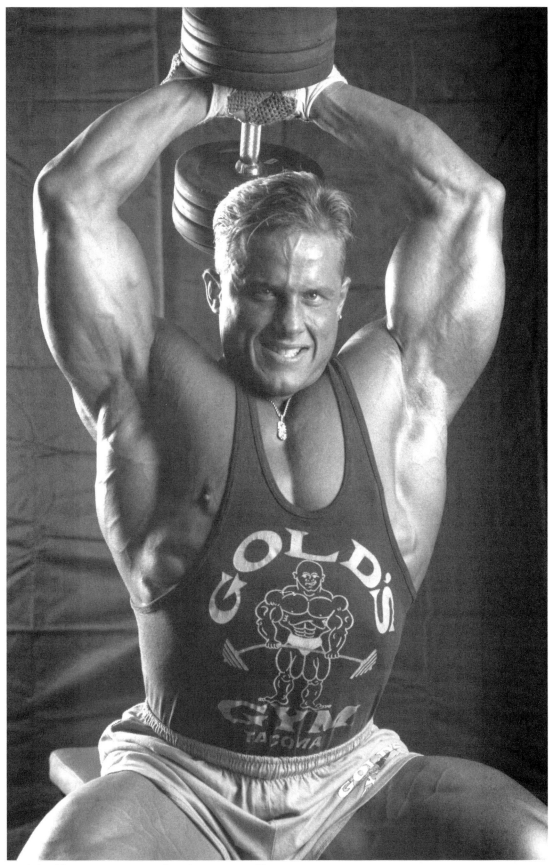

Bodybuilder Craig Titus. *Photo by Irvin J. Gelb.*

Carbohydrates. Carbohydrate is the body's preferred fuel source during exercise. It is stored in the liver and muscles as glycogen. More than 99 percent of the carbohydrates you eat are used by the body to make adenosine triphosphate (ATP). This is a molecular fuel used by the muscles to power contractions. The more carbohydrates you include in your diet, the better your muscles run.

In 1967 a classic study examined the effects of carbohydrate intake on glycogen levels and endurance. Endurance was measured by exercise time to exhaustion, with the subjects training at 75 percent of their maximal aerobic capacity.

The researchers found a direct relationship between carbohydrate content of the diet and endurance time. A low-carbohydrate diet (5 percent of calories) provided enough muscle glycogen stores to sustain 60 minutes of exercise. A moderate-carbohydrate diet (50 percent of calories) resulted in glycogen levels to sustain 115 minutes of exercise. The high-carbohydrate diet (82 percent of calories) supported 170 minutes of high-intensity exercise. Clearly, a high-carbohydrate diet is beneficial for endurance.[1]

The best sources of carbohydrates to meet the energy demands of the body are starchy carbs and fibrous carbs. I recommend that you eat at least one or two servings of starchy carbs and one or two servings of fibrous carbs at each meal, along with a lean-protein source.

High-fiber foods such as fibrous carbs contain the many types of fiber required for good health. Among these are gums, found in plants; pectin, the "cement" that holds the cell walls of plants together in plant tissues; mucilage, a protein/carbohydrate substance; lignin, a constituent of plant cells that holds them together; and cellulose, a plant carbohydrate that provides bulk to help with elimination.

Fiber and protein slow the digestion of starchy carbs, resulting in a gradual release of glucose into the bloodstream and more sustained energy levels. This is in contrast to the sharp surge triggered by simple and refined sugars. When you combine lean proteins, starchy carbohydrates, and fibrous carbs in meals, you have more energy, better glycogen reserves, and less fat storage.

Fat. After meeting your daily protein and carbohydrate requirements, be sure to include a certain amount of fat in your diet. Good sources are safflower oil, sunflower oil, linseed oil, and flaxseed oil. These dietary fats provide essential fatty acids and help the body absorb fat-soluble vitamins such as vitamin A, vitamin D, and vitamin E. I recommend that you eat up to one tablespoon a day of EFAs.

Even though fat is a highly concentrated source of energy, it can't be metabolized fast enough to meet the energy requirements of intense exercise. It takes 30 to 60 minutes of exercise for fatty acids to be available to the muscles for fuel. Not only that, more oxygen is needed to burn fat than to burn carbohydrates—another reason why carbs are the body's preferred fuel.

Despite this, some bodybuilders and athletes have experimented with high-fat diets. With the exception of nutrition programs using MCT oil, these diets can be dangerous for several reasons. While being high in fat, they are also low in carbohydrates. Low-carbohydrate diets can upset the body's electrolyte balance, namely the sodium/potassium ratio.

The fats typically used in high-fat, non–MCT oil diets come from processed sources, often containing high levels of bacteria, which impair the function of the reticuloendothelial system (RES). One of the most important functions of the RES is that it clears harmful bacteria from the system. But when a person goes on a high-fat diet for any length of time, antibody-producing cells in the RES become clogged with fat droplets, and their ability to purge bacteria is reduced. Bacteria goes undigested, without being processed by the liver, and can end up in the lungs, causing inflammation and possible organ failure. Clearly, it's vital to moderate your intake of dietary fat.

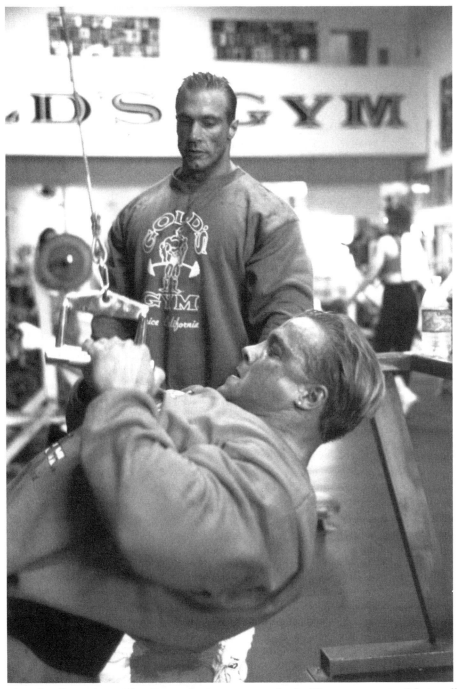

1993 Nationals Champion Mike Francois (top) spots Craig Titus on a set of lat pulldowns. *Photo by Irvin J. Gelb.*

7 SUPPLEMENTAL NUTRITION FOR AEROBIC ENERGY

Many of the bodybuilders I work with include up to two hours a day of aerobics—in addition to daily weight-training workouts—in their training programs. This intense level of training requires fuel from the proper foods, eaten in the right combinations. Along with food, certain supplements can help optimize the body's energy systems to meet higher intensity demands. Here are some recommendations for supplementation if you want to work out harder and longer, with more energy.

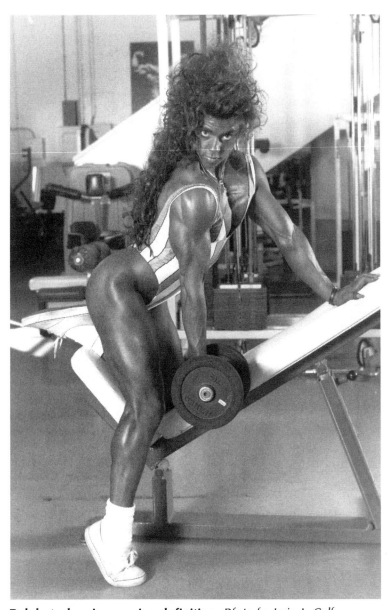

Michele Ann Ralabate has impressive definition. *Photo by Irvin J. Gelb.*

Branched-Chain Amino Acids. Unless you properly fuel yourself with quality calories, high-intensity aerobics can result in the loss of lean body mass. Endurance activities, for example, cause loss of lean tissue because as fat and carbohydrate fuels are exhausted, the body draws on its own muscle tissue to use as fuel.

The so-called branched-chain amino acids (leucine, isoleucine, and valine) are unique in that they can also be used directly as fuel by the muscles. Branched-chain amino acid supplements should always be taken with meals (two per meal), because they need insulin from carbohydrates to be transported into the muscles for growth and repair.

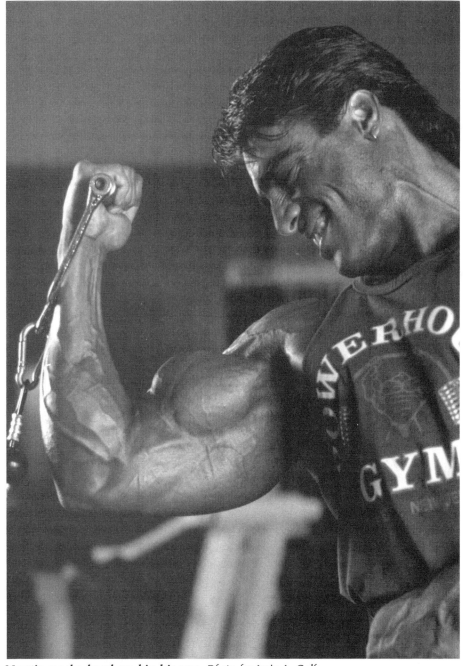

Jimmy Mentis works hard on his biceps. *Photo by Irvin J. Gelb.*

Aspartates. Have you ever noticed an ammonia smell in your clothes after a hard workout? This occurs because your body was using some amino acids as fuel but was not able to clear the waste products efficiently. When this happens, the carbon skeleton of amino acids is burned, leaving ammonia as a by-product.

Ammonia is converted to urea in a metabolic process called the "urea cycle," which prepares it to be excreted in the urine. The urea cycle requires certain chemical compounds called "aspartates," which are available in supplement form. This supplement works by providing nutrients that are used by the body to detoxify the waste products of protein catabolism and to filter out the waste products generated during intense training. By eliminating these waste products, you have more energy to train. Ammonia is very toxic and will stop energy production in the cell. Using aspartates to neutralize the ammonia as soon as it forms gives you more energy and endurance.

Aspartate supplements are usually formulated with other nutrients that optimize energy production. Among them are inosine for improved oxygen utilization, ferulic acid for better recovery and workout capacity, l-phenylalanine for mental concentration, and d-phenylalanine for an elevated pain threshold. I recommend that bodybuilders and athletes take aspartate-containing supplements on an empty stomach about 30 to 60 minutes before training.

Liver Tablets. Perhaps the most crucial supplement for bodybuilders engaged in an intense aerobics program is desiccated liver. I can't overemphasize the importance of this supplement. What is aerobic activity all about anyway? It involves producing energy over an extended period of time. Liver tablets help by providing heme iron, protein, and B-complex vitamins.

Iron is essential for the manufacture of two important proteins in the body: hemoglobin, a constituent of red blood cells that gives them their color; and myoglobin, an oxygen-carrying protein in muscle cells. Hemoglobin picks up oxygen from the lungs and transports it to the body's cells, where it is used to produce energy from the foods you eat. Myoglobin allows oxygen to be consumed inside muscle cells. Without adequate iron, the oxygen delivery system won't work, nor will oxygen be burned properly inside the cells. Clearly, iron has a central position in producing energy.

Although the body usually has good stores of iron, deficiencies are common. As many as 22 percent of American women are iron-deficient, often because of excessively heavy periods, pregnancy, or poor diets. The daily iron requirement for women is 18 mg, but on average they obtain only 10 to 12 mg.[1] Because men have lower daily iron requirements, they are somewhat less vulnerable to deficiencies. Many times a feeling of fatigue or low energy is the result of an unrecognized iron deficiency.

Athletes have to be particularly careful. About 10 percent of male athletes and 22 to 25 percent of female athletes are iron-deficient.[2] Deficiencies can occur with aerobics and endurance training. These deficiencies can actually destroy red blood cells rather than build them up—if nutrition is faulty. If you want to recover and be stronger as a result of your workout, you have to feed your body with the iron and protein it needs to make red blood cells.

Dietary sources of iron are classified as either "heme" iron or "nonheme" iron. Heme iron is chemically bound to heme—the component of hemoglobin that is responsible for its ability to carry oxygen in red blood cells. Heme also gives these cells their color.

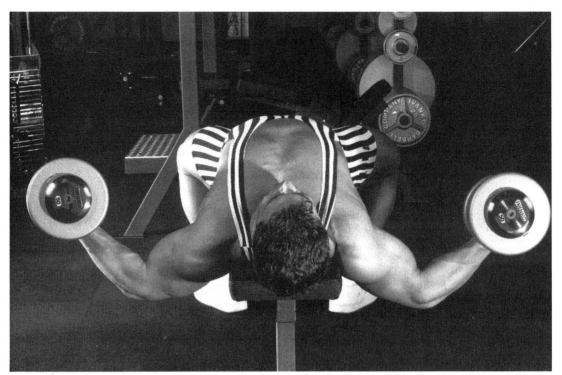
Supplements increase the nutrient density of your diet so you can train harder and longer. *Photo by Irvin J. Gelb.*

Good sources of heme iron are red meat and liver. White-meat chicken and turkey breast also contain heme iron but in lower amounts. The advantage of heme iron is that it's very well absorbed by the body. About 15 to 20 percent of the iron in red meat and liver is taken up. The problem with these foods, however, is their high fat and cholesterol content. This is why desiccated liver tablets, which are defatted and contain almost no cholesterol, are excellent sources of readily absorbed heme iron.

Plants have a different form of iron, one that is not bound to heme, and it's called "nonheme" iron. The body doesn't absorb nonheme iron as well as it does heme iron. Less than 2 percent of the iron in spinach is absorbed, for example.

In addition to providing heme iron, desiccated liver tablets supply extra protein. As I discussed earlier in section #5, on protein and muscular hardness, sports anemia can be caused by aerobic exercise. Contrary to what its name suggests, sports anemia is associated not with a true iron deficiency but rather with inadequate protein. The body starts to use red blood cells to make myoglobin and draws on red blood cells and blood proteins to get protein for muscular repair.

Desiccated liver tablets also contain B-complex vitamins. This vitamin group is active in converting carbohydrates into glucose, which the body burns to produce energy. B-complex vitamins are also involved in the metabolism of fats and proteins.

For best results, I recommend that you take several liver tablets with each meal. Along with ample calories from high-density foods, desiccated liver supplements should help you reach peak levels of performance, growth, and recovery.

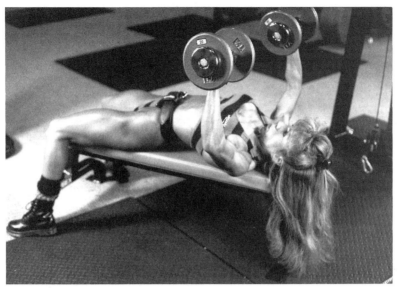

Endurance and stamina are critical for intense workouts. *Photo by Irvin J. Gelb.*

Carbohydrate Supplements. For a supplemental source of carbohydrate, choose a product that contains rice dextrin or maltodextrin, complex carbohydrates made from grain. Maltodextrin has been found to be the ideal carbohydrate source for replenishing glycogen reserves. It's digested and absorbed more rapidly than conventional carbs from food, but not so fast that it causes an overrelease of insulin and subsequent fat production. Maltodextrin provides a much more uniform energy level than do simple sugars. This type of supplement can be taken before, during, and after workouts for best results.

MCT Oil. Medium-chain triglyceride oil (MCT oil), also known as medium-chain fatty acid oil (MCFA oil), provides twice the energy of protein and carbohydrate (8.3 calories per gram for MCT oil versus 4 calories per gram for carbs and protein) and is absorbed into the bloodstream as rapidly as glucose. MCT oil is preferentially used as fuel for energy, instead of being stored by the body. As an added benefit, MCT oil has a "thermogenic" effect, which means that it is converted to energy very rapidly. It's an extremely concentrated source of calories that is rapidly absorbed and metabolized for energy by the body. I like to think of MCT oil as human jet fuel.

Another key point is that some of the energy from MCT oil is converted by the liver into ketone bodies, which are used as easily as glucose for fuel by the muscles. The efficiency of utilization of ketones as fuel improves as the body adapts to MCT oil. In other words, your body gets better at using this supplement as it gets accustomed to it. Thus, using it consistently will allow you to get more out of it when you really need it. In addition, these same ketone bodies produced by MCT oil help prevent the use of the amino acids as fuel. That way, your aminos get used as protein to build muscle instead of being burned for energy.

Start with a half tablespoon of MCT oil at every meal. After a few days, increase to one tablespoon with each meal. During hard training, many athletes go as high as two or three tablespoons per meal—a level they have found to be beneficial.

8 RECOVERY: A CONDITION FOR GROWTH

To achieve maximum muscular growth from your workouts, you must create conditions that allow your muscles to recover. "Recovery" refers to mechanisms that resupply the muscles with nutrients and cleanse them of waste products so that the body can properly rebuild itself after a workout. Your muscles have four requirements for optimum recovery: glycogen restoration, aerobics, electrolyte repletion, and rest.

Glycogen Restoration. Glycogen is carbohydrate stored in the liver and muscles. The longer you exercise, the lower your glycogen reserves become. Those reserves can continue to fall over a period of days if you're not consuming enough carbohydrates in your diet. As a result, you feel fatigued—a feeling that is often interpreted as "overtraining." I call it "undereating." By that, I mean insufficient nutrition.

How much carbohydrate should you eat to avoid this condition? We now know that diets providing 500 to 600 grams of carbohydrate a day provide complete repletion of glycogen stores and let you maintain a heavy training schedule.

Your individual carbohydrate requirements depend largely on the type, intensity, duration, and frequency of your exercise. The longer and harder you train, the more carbohydrates you will need. If you fail to get a good pump while working out, you are probably glycogen-deficient. (For additional recommendations on how to maximize your glycogen reserves, see the next section on supercompensation.) Muscles are most receptive to synthesizing new glycogen within the first few hours following exercise. Consuming the proper kinds of carbohydrates in solid or beverage form immediately after a workout assists in glycogen restoration.

Aerobics. Aerobic exercise has many fitness benefits, namely cardiovascular conditioning and fat-burning. There's another benefit as well: Aerobic exercise expands your network of capillaries. These are the body's smallest blood vessels, and they allow water, glucose, amino acids, and other materials to be absorbed through their walls to body tissues. This expansion of capillaries is called "cardiovascular density."

Think of cardiovascular density as a highly efficient pickup-and-delivery system. With good cardiovascular density, there are more blood vessels to supply body tissues with the nutrients required for energy production and the raw materials needed for growth, maintenance, and repair. In addition, waste products, particularly carbon dioxide produced when food is burned with oxygen for energy, can be cleared away much more effectively. To build cardiovascular density and ultimately optimize your recovery, include hard, intense aerobics in your training program—at least several times a week, for approximately 45 to 60 minutes each session.

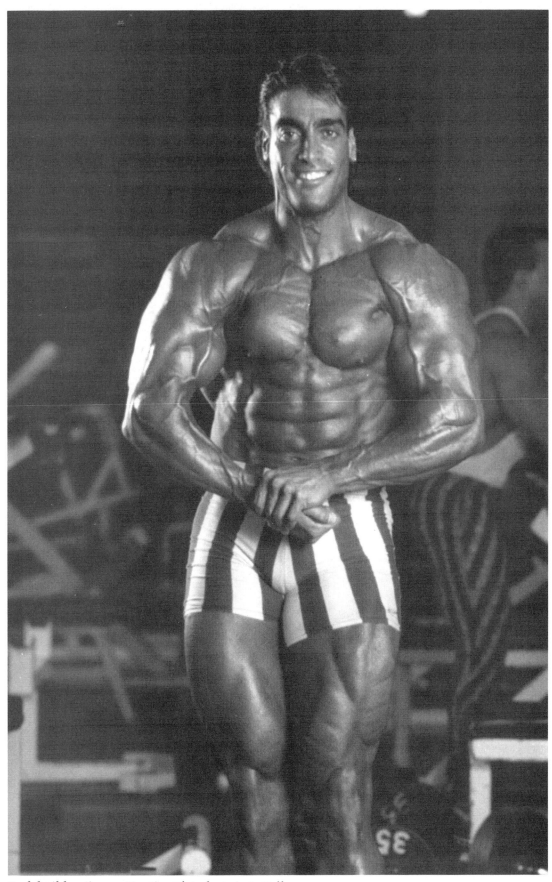

Bodybuilder Jimmy Mentis. *Photo by Irvin J. Gelb.*

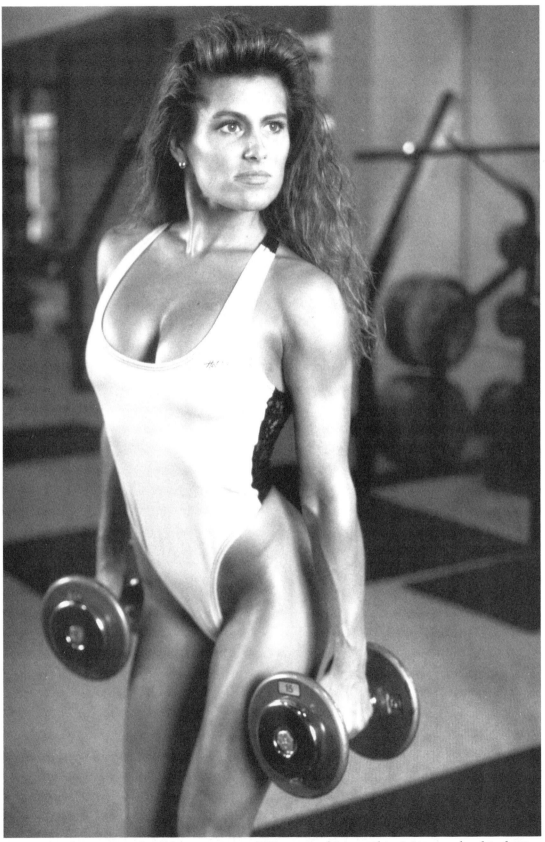

Hope Lane is an example of how proper nutrition, aerobics, and training can lead to better shape and overall fitness. *Photo by Irvin J. Gelb.*

Electrolytes. Bodybuilders who train all out must pay closer attention to minerals and electrolytes. Hard, intense training, particularly during the summer months, can deplete these needed nutrients from the body through perspiration and normal metabolic processes.

Found in fish, poultry, and vegetables, electrolytes are minerals that are responsible for maintaining the body's fluid balance, both inside and outside cells. Fluids protect internal organs, supply nutrients and oxygen to cells and tissues for growth and repair, and transport carbon dioxide and other waste products away from cells.

The main electrolytes in extracellular fluid are sodium, calcium, and chloride; in the intracellular fluid, they are potassium, magnesium, and phosphorus. These nutrients provide a life-sustaining environment for all body cells and must be kept in proper balance for optimum health.

In addition to their electrolytic functions, these minerals play other vital roles in the body. Calcium, for example, is required for the formation of body structures, particularly bones and teeth. It's the most abundant mineral in the body, with about 99 percent deposited in bones. It's important to mention that dietary calcium is not well absorbed. In fact, only about 20 to 30 percent of the calcium you get from foods is absorbed, making mineral-electrolyte supplementation a good idea.

The next most abundant mineral in the body is phosphorus. This mineral is essential for the formation of body structures, muscular contractions, nerve transmission, and kidney function. Phosphorus also plays a key role in energy production.

Magnesium is required for the metabolism of protein and carbohydrates. This mineral depends on the presence of calcium for its action. So when selecting a mineral-electrolyte supplement, make sure that the magnesium is equal to or at least 70 percent of the calcium.

Another essential mineral is chloride. As an electrolyte, chloride helps maintain the pressure that causes fluids to pass in and out of cells until an equilibrium is reached on both sides of the cell membrane.

Potassium is required for nerve transmission, muscular contraction, and glycogen storage. It's also involved in the synthesis of protein. Potassium works together with sodium to regulate fluid balance. Even though sodium has a bad reputation because of its link to high blood pressure and heart disease, some sodium is needed by the body for good health.

The trick is to keep your sodium/potassium ratio in balance. By eating natural carbohydrates, you take in high amounts of potassium. If there's too little sodium in your system, your body accelerates its production of aldosterone, a hormone that regulates the vital sodium/potassium balance. Inadequate concentrations of sodium can actually make you look smooth, rather than defined.

As you can tell, there are many issues surrounding the intake of mineral-electrolytes. It's a good idea to take a balanced mineral-electrolyte formulation with your meals to ensure that you're replenishing your body with adequate amounts of these vital nutrients.

Rest. The main time muscle grows is during rest and sleep. Additionally, growth hormone (GH), which regulates growth, increases to maximum levels during sleep. Suffice to say, you need adequate rest and sleep as conditions for growth. But how much? Requirements vary from individual to individual.

You might need eight hours of sleep, while someone else might need only six. The key is to be consistent, going to bed at the same time every night and getting up at the same time. Split routines, in which portions of the body are worked on different days, provide adequate rest and recuperation for muscles.

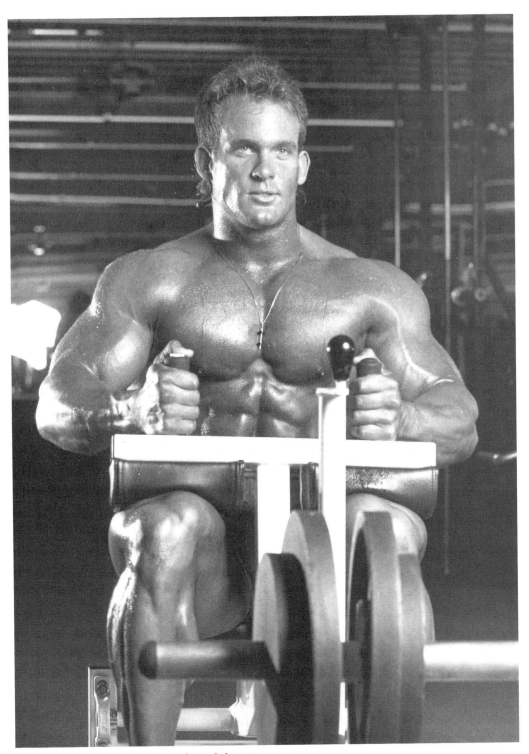

Bodybuilder John DePolo. *Photo by Ralph DeHaan.*

9 SUPERCOMPENSATION: GREATER STAMINA FOR HARDER TRAINING

Want to double the amount of glycogen stored in your muscles for extra stamina? Then try "supercompensation," a technique borrowed from endurance athletes and adapted for bodybuilders. Endurance athletes do it like this: For three days, they train as usual but eat a low-carbohydrate diet to deplete glycogen reserves. They rest for the next three days and consume a high-carbohydrate diet. During this rest period, the body overcompensates and stores more glycogen in the muscles than usual.

You can use a similar approach. But as a bodybuilder, you shouldn't empty your glycogen reserves completely, because you could lose precious muscle. As a general guideline, I suggest that while lowering carbs, you adjust your carbohydrate intake so that you lose your pump about three-fourths of the way through your workout. For most bodybuilders, this turns out to be between 100 and 300 grams of carbs per day—an amount sufficient to stimulate supercompensation without causing muscle loss. (Supplementation with branched-chain amino acids may help prevent muscle protein from being burned for energy.) After a few days of lowering your carb intake, gradually increase it to 500 to 600 grams to reload your muscles with glycogen.

Along with adjustments in diet, include regular aerobics in your training schedule. Aerobic exercise, like endurance training, stimulates the manufacture of muscle glycogen by accelerating the activity of an enzyme responsible for glycogen storage. This effect occurs after exercise and is localized in the muscles used. In other words, aerobic training such as running or cycling, which targets the legs, promotes glycogen loading in legs but not in the other parts of the body.

To better restock glycogen throughout your body, organize your aerobic session into "cross-training" segments: 20 to 25 minutes on a stationary cycle or stair-climbing machine to stimulate glycogen storage in the legs, followed by 20 to 25 minutes on a rowing machine for the arms and upper body.

Starchy carbohydrates are the preferred food choice for replenishing glycogen. Unlike simple sugars, complex carbs are released into the bloodstream more slowly. This slow release maintains elevation of insulin, a hormone, which, among its other jobs, stimulates the action of glycogen-storage enzymes.

As mentioned earlier, maltodextrin-based supplements provide an excellent source of carbohydrates. But how well does maltodextrin work as a fuel for supercompensation? At least one study has looked into this, and the results are promising.[1]

The athletes in this study depleted their carbohydrates for three days by cutting carbs down to just 20 percent of their total intake, while they continued to train. The next three days, to rebuild glycogen, they upped their carbs to 90 percent of their diet and reduced their training levels slightly. One group loaded up with rice and pasta; the other, with a maltodextrin-based beverage. Afterward, the researchers took muscle biopsies of each athlete.

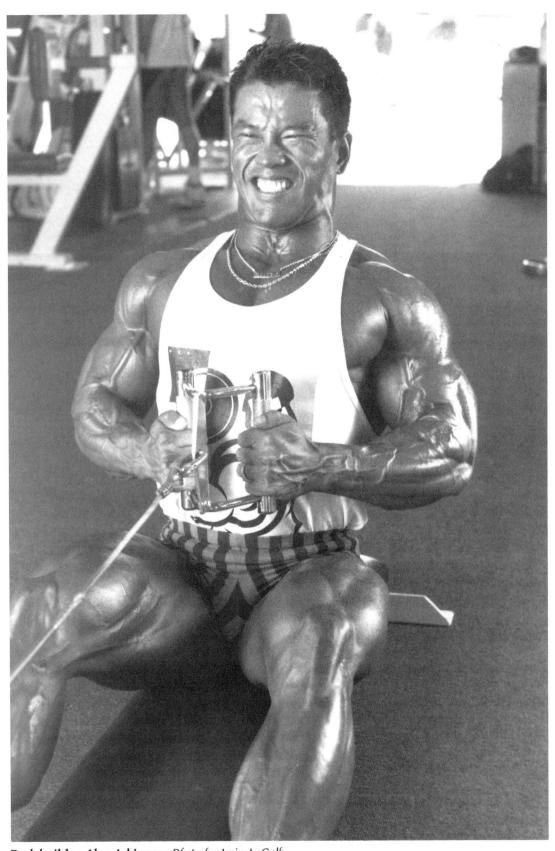

Bodybuilder Alan Ichinose. *Photo by Irvin J. Gelb.*

As it turned out, the athletes on maltodextrin stored more glycogen than the athletes who ate rice and pasta. The reason, said researchers, was that maltodextrin in liquid form may be better absorbed and used by the body.

A maltodextrin-based supplement has another advantage: It's the perfect post-workout carbohydrate. Glycogen storage is maximized when you consume carbohydrates immediately after exercise. But like a lot of people, you might not be hungry then. Take a maltodextrin beverage instead of solid food. It's less filling and will answer your muscles' need for carbohydrate.

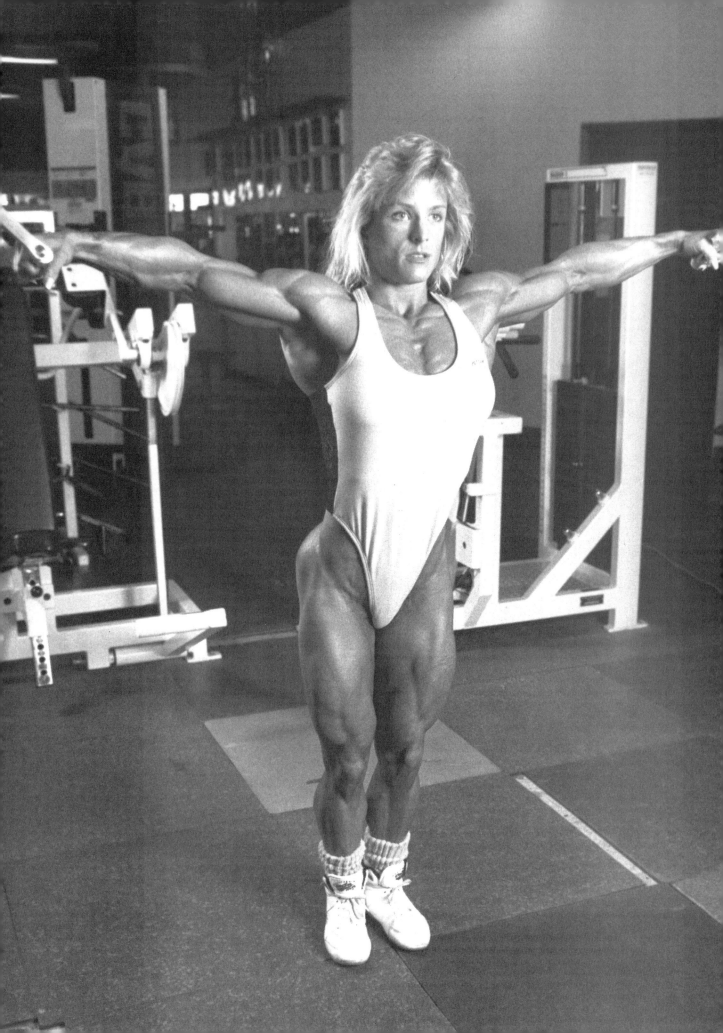

PART
II
TRAINING
SECRETS

Bodybuilder Sue Price. *Photo by Irvin J. Gelb.*

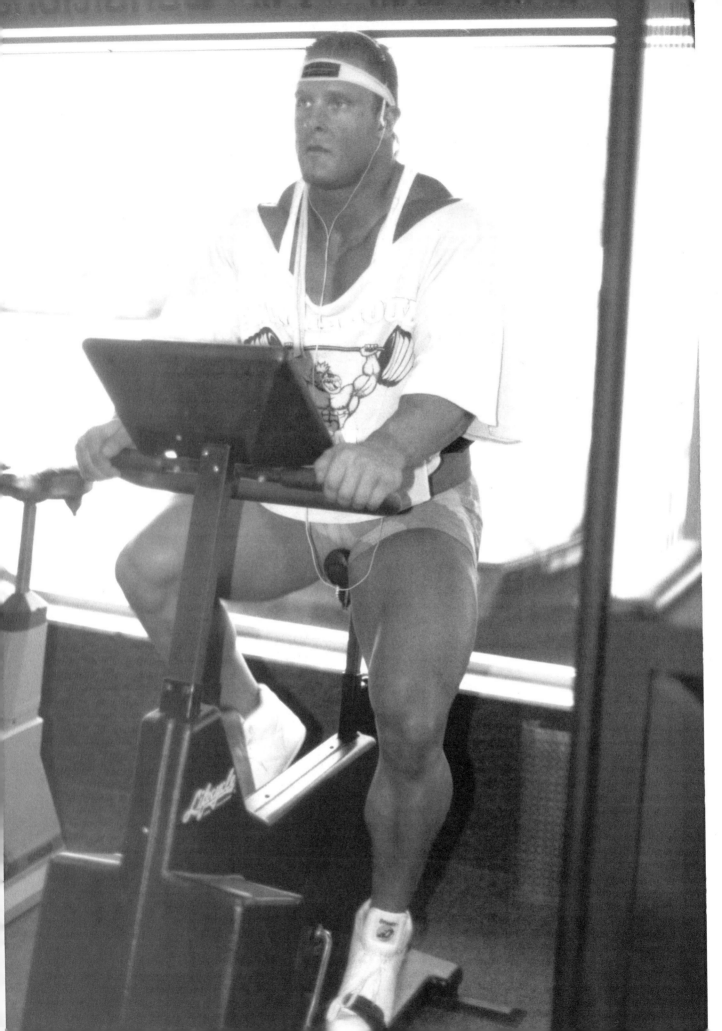

10 GENERAL CARDIOVASCULAR CONDITIONING: BOOST YOUR FAT-BURNING CAPACITY

A critical shift in thinking about aerobics is in order. For a long time now, exercisers have been urged to achieve their "target heart rate" during aerobic activity. This is the elevation of the pulse to approximately 60 to 80 percent of your maximum heart rate (220 heartbeats per minute minus your age). Reaching target heart rate and keeping it there for at least 20 minutes is supposed to boost general cardiovascular conditioning. It's also always been assumed that if you exercise at your target heart rate long enough, you burn fat.

Optimal cardiovascular conditioning is not achieved by just raising your target heart rate, however. It's achieved by increasing your "oxygen uptake," or VO_{2max}. This represents your body's maximum capability to deliver oxygen to the working muscles. So how do you boost your VO_{2max}? By exercising so intensely that you're breathing hard. The harder you breathe, the more energy you expend, and the more fat you burn because you're doing more work.

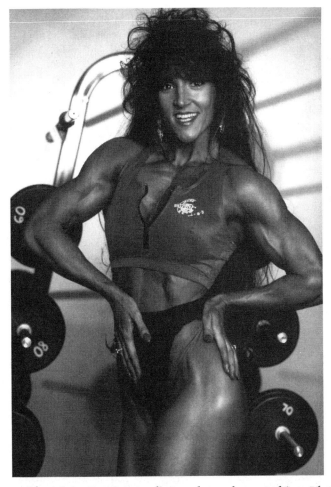

Lisa Lorio gets lean with strict attention to diet and regular aerobics. *Photo by Jimmie D. King.*

Intense aerobics enhance cardiovascular fitness, boost your fat-burning potential, and drive your recovery mechanisms. *Photo by Irvin J. Gelb.*

Train consistently like this, and some important metabolic changes take place inside the body. First, the mitochondria (cellular furnaces where fat and other nutrients are burned) increase in size and total number inside muscle fibers. Second, muscle fibers build up more aerobic enzymes—special chemicals involved in fat-burning. Third, aerobic exercise appears to increase levels of myoglobin, a muscle compound that accelerates the transfer of oxygen from the bloodstream into the muscle fibers.

Larger mitochondria and more of them, greater levels of aerobic enzymes, and increased blood flow—these factors all boost the fat-burning capability of muscle fibers. The more aerobically fit you become, the more your body learns to burn fat for energy. So you can see why aerobic exercise is so important for leaning out.

Endurance athletes have known these things all along. That's why bodybuilders can learn a lot from the training regimens of endurance athletes. They train regularly and at long durations at near VO_{2max}. As a result, their muscles are conditioned to rely more heavily on fat for energy and less on stored carbohydrate (glycogen). To approach the training level of an endurance athlete, perform aerobics several times a week, for 45 to 60 minutes each time. But don't "coast." Work out hard, so that you're breathing hard. The harder you breathe, the more fat you burn.

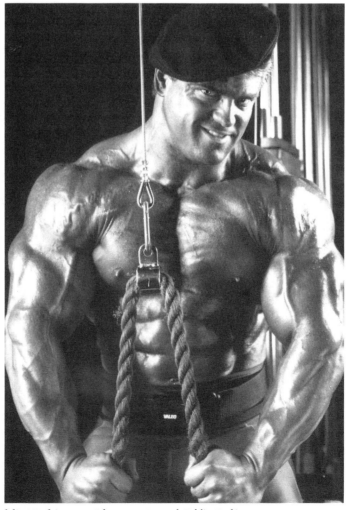

"Major Guns" Eddie Robinson. *Photo courtesy of Eddie Robinson.*

11 SPECIFIC CARDIOVASCULAR CONDITIONING: MORE POWER TO SUSTAIN MUSCULAR CONTRACTIONS

Do your muscles "burn" too early in a set, forcing you to cut your reps short? If so, you need to build your "specific cardiovascular conditioning." This describes the ability of your muscles to take in and use oxygen, required for energy production, and to efficiently clear the waste products of exercise from the muscles. The better your specific cardiovascular conditioning, the longer you can contract your muscles before you feel the burning sensation—and the harder you can push each set.

The burn is the result of a biochemical reaction to anaerobic (without oxygen) exercise like weight training. As you work out, the glycogen stored in your muscles is turned into glucose, which is then broken down into a chemical called pyruvate. It combines with oxygen and converts to carbon dioxide and water. These are expelled as waste gases during breathing.

If oxygen is in short supply, as often happens when you work out beyond your aerobic capacity, pyruvate turns into lactic acid. Lactic acid builds up in the muscle, producing the burn. It becomes harder for the muscles to contract. Fatigue sets in. Lots of lactic acid in the muscle can stop contractions entirely.

These responses subside as soon as oxygen is resupplied, usually during the rest periods between sets. Most of the lactic acid is rapidly changed back into pyruvate and finally to carbon dioxide and water.

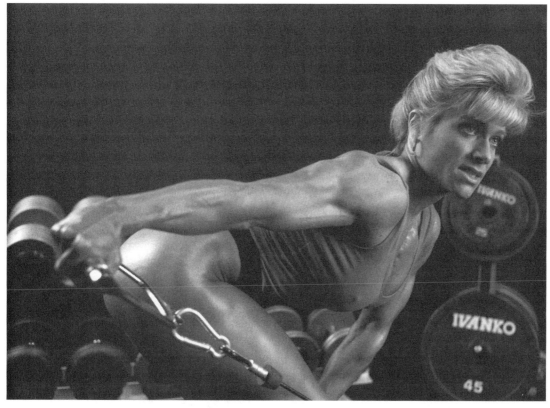

Perfect muscularity. *Photo by Ralph DeHaan.*

Well-trained muscles—those with good specific cardiovascular conditioning—can keep going because lactic acid and other waste products are being efficiently cleared. Naturally, this is desirable, since you perform more reps and sets without stopping.

How do you build specific cardiovascular density? Primarily by forcing the muscles to do more work. After your pyramid sets (a technique of increasing poundages from set to set), perform 3 or 4 "exhaustion sets," high-rep sets with lower poundages. These sets develop specific cardiovascular density. On each exhaustion set, aim for 20 to 30 repetitions.

One of the best techniques for building specific cardiovascular conditioning during the exhaustion set portion of a routine is descending sets. Descending sets are the opposite of pyramid sets. You start with a weight with which you can get at least 30 reps and then reduce that poundage on subsequent sets.

Take the biceps curl, for example. Load the barbell up with a weight light enough to let you do 30 reps to failure. Rest and then reduce the poundage by about 25 percent. Go for 25 reps or to failure on your second set. Rest and reduce the weight again by 25 percent for another high-rep set performed to failure. Continue in this manner until you're unable to perform any more reps.

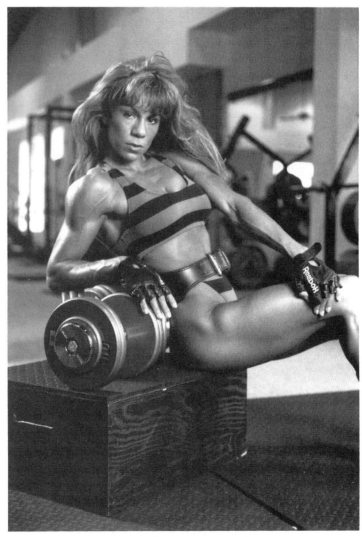

Lisa Ibarra—a model of fitness and good health. *Photo by Irvin J. Gelb.*

12 TRAIN YOUR MUSCLES TO BURN MORE FAT

Can weight training ever be viewed as a fat-burning activity? Definitely. And the reason has to do with muscle fibers, the basic component of the muscle. Muscle fibers are divided into three types: slow-twitch (also called slow-oxidative—SO—or Type I), fast-twitch oxidative-glycolytic (FOG or Type IIa), and pure fast-twitch (FT or Type IIb).

The slow-twitch fibers contract slowly. But they can sustain their contractions for long periods, without fatiguing. These fibers are used more in endurance activities such as long-distance running or swimming. Genetically, athletes with a predominance of slow-twitch fibers perform well in endurance competition.

Slow-twitch fibers get most of their energy from burning fat, a process that requires oxygen. This process is further kindled by the fibers' ample supply of blood vessels, mitochondria, and glycogen and blood fats inside their cells.

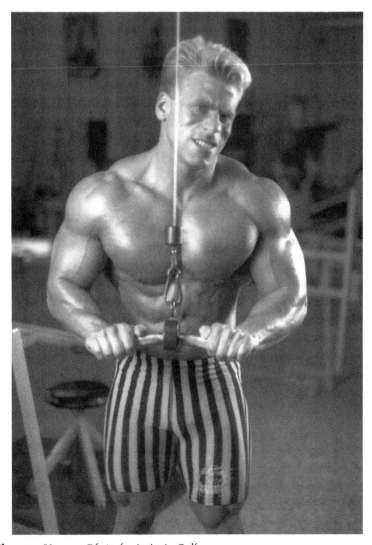

Bodybuilder Thomas Varga. *Photo by Irvin J. Gelb.*

The pure fast-twitch fibers are different. They contract rapidly but fatigue more easily. Their energy comes from burning glycogen. There are fewer mitochondria in the cellular makeup of fast-twitch fibers. Athletes who excel in speed or power events such as sprinting or weight lifting appear to have a higher percentage of fast-twitch fibers.

Fast-twitch oxidative-glycolytic fibers contract quickly, too, but they don't fatigue as fast. This may be because they have more mitochondria than the pure fast-twitch type but less than the slow-twitch fibers. But like the slow-twitch variety, fat can be burned by the fast-twitch oxidative fibers for energy.

Interestingly, you can change pure fast-twitch fibers into fast-twitch oxidative by performing hard, long-duration aerobics or intense, high-repetition training. Furthermore, this type of training actually increases the number of mitochondria in fast-twitch fibers to levels higher than those found in slow-twitch fibers.[1] With more mitochondria in muscle cells, the fast-twitch muscle fibers burn more fat. Through highly intense training, your body literally becomes a fat-burning machine.

If you want to burn more body fat, I suggest that you do high-rep work using heavy poundages. Work out intensely—so that you're breathing hard each time you finish a set. Increase the frequency and duration of your aerobics, too.

This regimen is precisely how competitive bodybuilders train to lose fat before a contest. It's an all-out approach that verges on overtraining. But that's what you have to do to change the fat-burning capacity of your muscle fibers.

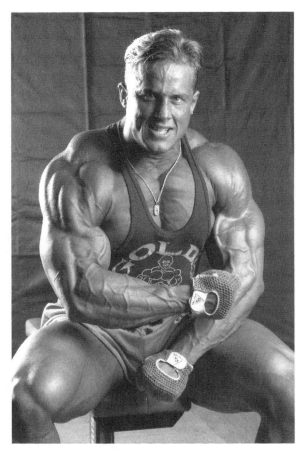

Massive Craig Titus. *Photo by Irvin J. Gelb.*

13 REGULATING GROWTH BY EXERCISE AND NUTRITION

Along with nutrition, exercise is one of the best ways to control the fat-burning and muscle-building actions of certain hormones produced by the body, namely adrenaline, testosterone, and growth hormone (GH).

To illustrate how these hormones help you lose body fat, let's start with adrenaline. When you work out, adrenaline is released, and it heads directly to fat cells. There, it sparks a chemical reaction, activating a special enzyme that breaks down stored fat into fatty acids. The fatty acids leave the fat cell, enter the bloodstream, and are carried to muscle cells to be used for energy.

Testosterone is a male hormone that seems to speed up the rate at which protein is used for muscle growth. Intense weight training triggers the production of testosterone. Concentrations in the blood start to climb, reaching peak levels 30 minutes into training. To take advantage of this increased testosterone level, you can perform highly intense training sessions using heavy, low-rep work for a duration of 30 to 60 minutes.

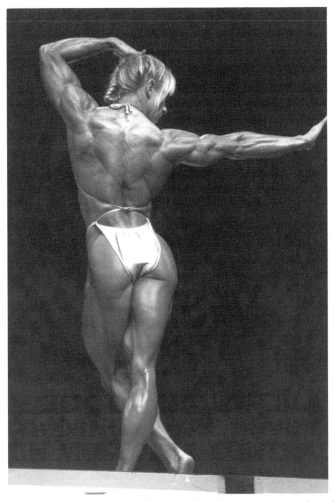

Note the muscular separation Denise Rutkowski displays onstage. *Photo by Irvin J. Gelb.*

Growth hormone (GH) is the most powerful growth-producing substance in the human body. Part of the reason is that GH helps ferry certain essential amino acids into muscle cells. GH also has a "lipolytic" effect, which means it mobilizes body fat from storage sites and increases its use for energy. GH is probably the most important hormone for bodybuilding because of its dual involvement in building muscle and burning fat.

There are several things you can do to naturally increase your GH levels. First, follow a diet that contains adequate protein (1.25 to 1.5 grams of protein per pound of body weight). A high-protein meal increases GH release.[1] Second, consider supplementing your diet with certain amino acids. The most effective oral combination for GH release is arginine pyroglutamate and lysine monohydrochloride. This is typically taken at bedtime and in the morning, always on an empty stomach. Glycine, another amino acid found in certain dietary supplements, is also a potent GH stimulator. The third way to increase your GH levels is to get enough sleep. GH is released at maximal levels during sleep.

Finally, train "smart." High-repetition work with moderate poundages has been shown in research to stimulate GH release. Given that heavy low-rep work maximizes testosterone release and high-rep work triggers GH release, you can design a routine that takes advantage of these hormonal processes.

For example, incorporate heavy pyramid sets and exhaustion sets into the same training session. Start with 1 or 2 warm-up sets with 15 reps each. Then select a poundage you can handle with proper form for 10 reps. Continue increasing the weight and do sets of 8, 6, and 4 reps. Next, decrease the weight and perform an exhaustion set of 20 reps to failure. Exhaustion sets help pump blood into the muscle and stimulate GH release.

14 STRETCHING FOR MASS AND MUSCULARITY

A special training technique I developed called "fascial stretching" can be incorporated into your training program to build strength and better develop the muscles. It strengthens and stretches the fascia, a thick, fibrous sheet of tissue that envelops individual muscles and groups of muscles and, like a divider, separates their layers and groupings. The fascia encloses other structures, too, including tendons, joints, blood vessels, nerves, and organs. The fascia functions like a shock absorber for the tissues it surrounds, protecting them from blows of athletics or the stresses of training and competition. On the molecular level, fascia tissue is stronger than structural steel.

To perform fascial stretching, you stretch between sets of weight-training exercises when the muscle is fully pumped (the pump has an additional stretch effect on the muscle). Special stretching exercises are used, several of which are explained below. Done consistently during workouts, fascial stretching stimulates muscular development and improves strength. The reason for this response is simple: When you stretch the fascia, you give the muscle underneath more room to grow. The result is larger muscles and better separation between muscle groups. I've seen this happen in working with athletes who use fascial stretching. What's more, I've observed that their strength levels can increase by as much as 20 percent.

There are other benefits as well. Stretching makes your body more flexible, giving your muscles and the joints they connect greater range of motion. A supple, flexible physique is less susceptible to injuries, because it can better withstand physical stresses. Stretching also helps prevent muscle soreness and promotes better recovery following training.

In addition, stretching loosens tight muscles, which tend to trap lactic acid, a waste product that accumulates in muscle cells during hard training. When lactic acid builds up, muscular fatigue is the result. Stretching helps release lactic acid from muscle cells into the bloodstream so that it does not interfere with muscular contraction. This loosening effect of stretching also helps you breathe better during workouts, increasing your oxygen utilization for improved energy levels.

Fascial stretching is not a gentle, touch-your-toes type of exercise you might associate with conventional stretching. As the stretch begins, the body part being trained is guided into position, stretched past the point of pain, and then held in that position for about 10 seconds. You should exhale and relax as you go into the stretch. Do not hold your breath.

Here are several fascial stretches for key parts of the body that you can integrate into your training program:

QUADRICEPS STRETCH

Start: Stand next to a bench or other piece of sturdy gym equipment. Bend your right knee. Holding your right ankle, bring your bent leg behind you. Position your ankle so that your instep is secured against the equipment. For balance, steady yourself by holding onto the equipment.

Stretch: Press your right heel to your buttocks while pushing your upper thigh down and back. Hold for 10 seconds, then release. Repeat with the left thigh. This stretch should be performed between sets of exercises that work the quadriceps, such as leg extensions or leg presses.

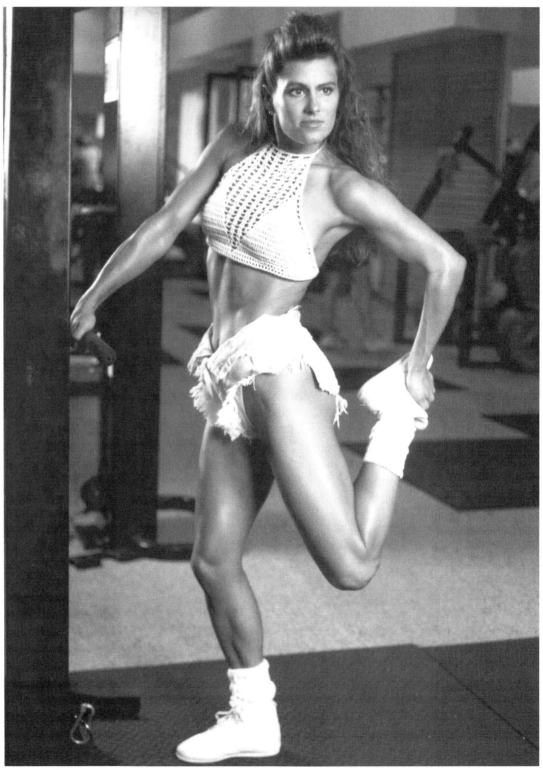

The quadriceps stretch should be performed between sets of leg exercises to improve muscular shape, size, and separation, as Hope Lane demonstrates. *Photo by Irvin J. Gelb.*

FORWARD HAMSTRING STRETCH

Start: To begin, sit with your legs extended straight out in front of you. Lean forward and clasp the tops of your feet. Make sure your knees are locked out tightly.

Stretch: Lean forward and pull the tops of your feet toward you, arching your back as hard as you can. Stretch hard. Hold for a count of 10 before releasing. Perform this stretch following sets of exercises such as leg curls.

SKIN-THE-CATS

Start: Skin-the-cat is a gymnastics-type movement that effectively stretches the pectoral muscles. It requires a great deal of practice and control. Take a medium (shoulder-width) overhand grip on the pull-up bar. Bend your knees and pull yourself up.

Stretch: Invert your body, pulling your feet in through the opening created by your hands. Then rotate around to a hanging position. On your way down, tuck your knees to your chest. At the completion of the movement, point your toes and try to touch the floor. You may want someone to help you through the movement. The entire stretch should be performed slowly, with full muscular control. Medium-grip skin-the-cats can be performed between sets of chest exercises such as bench presses or dumbbell flies.

Variations: A narrow grip (about twelve inches) will stretch the shoulders. As explained above, a shoulder-width grip with stretch the pecs. An even wider grip will stretch the biceps.

LAT STRETCH

Start: With both hands, grasp a bar or piece of stationary equipment. Place all the weight on the left side of your body—the side that will be stretched first. Cross your right leg over your left leg and step forward so that all your weight is on your left foot.

Stretch: Lean away from the bar, forming a comma with your body. With your left hand, push your shoulders in and through. Hold this position for 10 seconds. Repeat with the other side of your body. This stretch should be performed between sets of exercises that work the lats, such as lat pulldowns.

DELTOID STRETCH

Start: This stretch is performed at a bench press rack with a bar. Bend at the waist and take a wide grip on the bar. Your upper body should be parallel to the floor.

Stretch: Flex your lats and lower your shoulders down toward the floor as far as you can. Keep your arms tightly locked. Hold this position for a count of 10, then release. Perform the deltoid stretch between sets of overhead shoulder presses and other deltoid exercises.

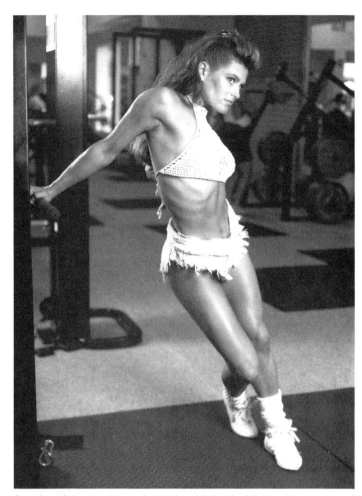

Hope Lane stretches her biceps. Stretches should be held for 10 seconds before releasing. *Photo by Irvin J. Gelb.*

BICEPS STRETCH

Start: Stand at arm's length from the bar, then grip the bar with your right hand.

Stretch: Rotate your torso as far to the left as you can. Hold for 10 seconds, then release. Repeat with the other arm. This is an excellent stretch to do between sets of biceps curls.

TRICEPS STRETCH

Start: Place your back against a bar or piece of stationary equipment. Hold on to the equipment and push your shoulder up against the bar. This pushes your triceps up. Bend your arms behind your head and point your elbows up toward the ceiling. Grasp your triceps with your other hand and pull it back. Bend your knees.

Stretch: To stretch your triceps, simply straighten your knees. Hold the stretched position for 10 seconds, then release. Perform this stretch between sets of any triceps exercise, including triceps pressdowns and triceps extensions.

15 A SPECIAL TRAINING SEQUENCE FOR RAPID RESULTS

Think about it: In most sports, the acts of training and competitive performance are one and the same. Runners run, swimmers swim, cyclists cycle, and so forth. Bodybuilders, however, are different. Their competitive performance happens only when they're onstage, posing in front of the judges and the audience.

If you want to improve in bodybuilding, you should train as other athletes do—by integrating performance (posing) with training. This goes for anyone who trains with weights: You don't have to be a competitive bodybuilder to pose. There are some advantages to posing during your workout. Let me explain by outlining a three-part training sequence:

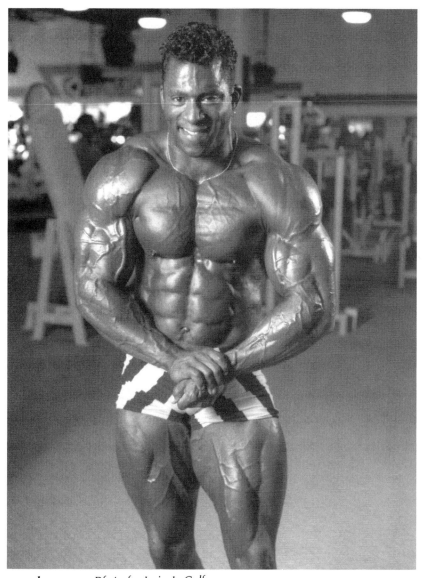

The most muscular pose. *Photo by Irvin J. Gelb.*

1. Do every exercise set as intensely as possible. This means overloading your muscles with more weight, more sets and repetitions, or both.
2. Follow each exercise set with the fascial stretch for the body part being worked. (Fascial stretching is my special method of stretching performed between each set and results in dramatic increases in mass, muscularity, muscular separation, and strength. See section #14 for instructions on how to perform fascial stretches.)
3. Pose the muscles being worked. Posing accentuates muscular hardness and separation. You have to think of it as a type of exercise. If you've never posed before, here are some instructions on how to correctly perform some key poses:

Front Double Biceps. Raise your arms up from your sides, to a point at which your upper arms form a straight line extended from your shoulders. Bend your elbows, make a fist, and flex your biceps hard. Keep your shoulders down and your elbows up so that your biceps are higher than your delts. Pull your lats out as you pose.

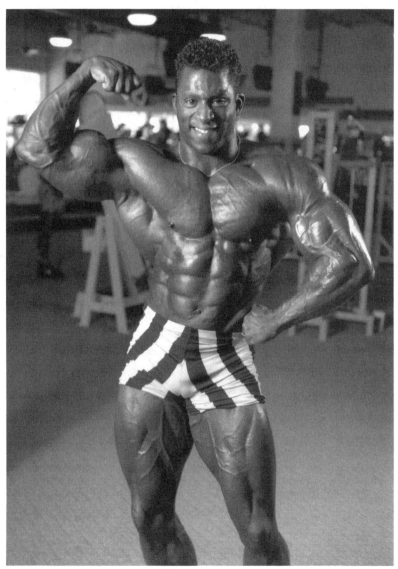

The front biceps pose. *Photo by Irvin J. Gelb.*

Front Lat Spread. Place your hands at your midsection and push your waist in. Press your shoulders down. Then pull your lats out and forward to make them visible from the front. Be sure to flex your quads at the same time.

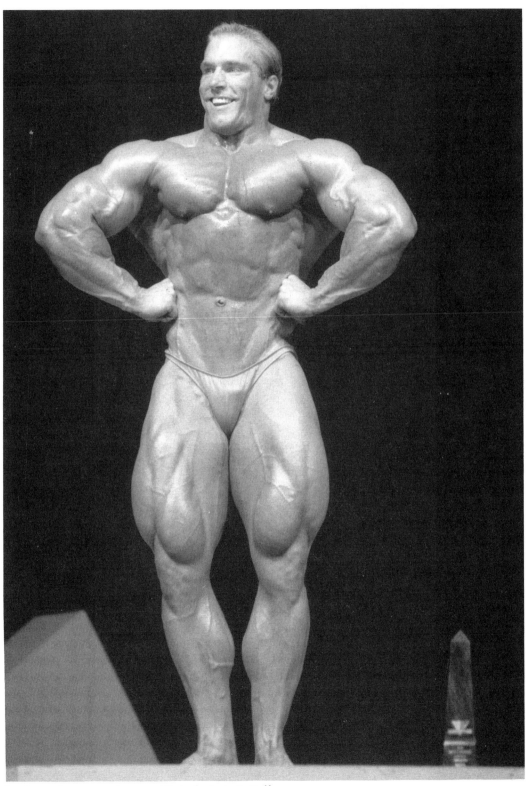

The front lat spread pose. *Photo by Irvin J. Gelb.*

Side Chest. For the best example of how to do this pose, look at pictures of Arnold Schwarzenegger in his competitive days. Notice how his chest was so elevated that the line created by his upper pecs was nearly parallel to the floor.

Clasp your hands in front. While keeping your rear shoulder down, push your sternum out and flex hard.

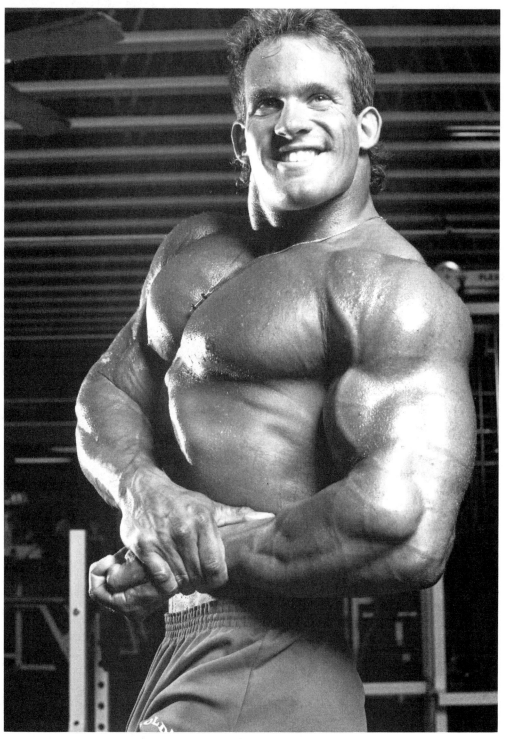

The side chest pose. *Photo by Irvin J. Gelb.*

Side Triceps. Position your legs with your inner thigh and calf pressed tightly against your rear leg. Keep your abs tight and pulled in. Clasp your hands behind you, in a cupped position. Don't clutch your wrist with your other hand. Rotate your upper body slightly to show the "V" that tapers up from your waist to your upper body.

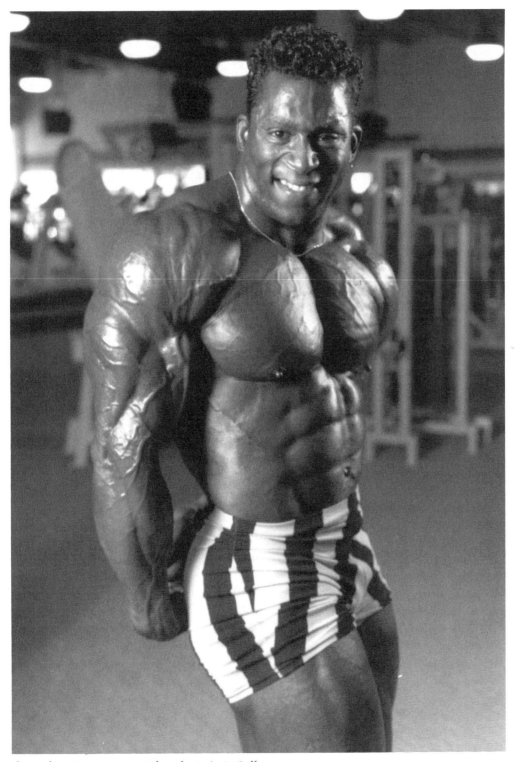

The side triceps pose. *Photo by Irvin J. Gelb.*

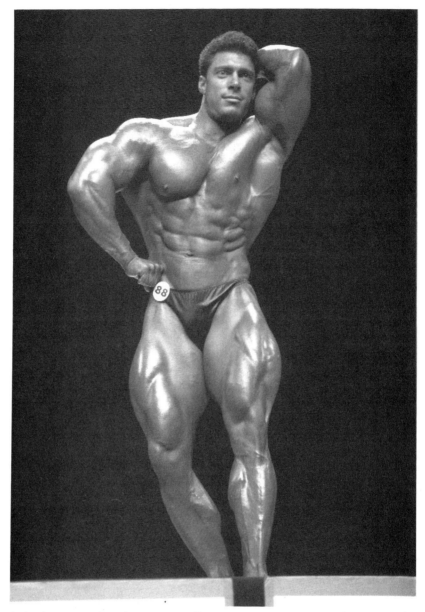

The ab and thigh pose. *Photo by Irvin J. Gelb.*

Ab and Thigh Pose. Start with your shoulders pressed down. Then bring them forward and flare your lats out. Keep your elbows up and back. Extend one leg out in front, angling it slightly. Naturally, you must flex that leg as tightly as possible so that every striation shows. In a coordinated fashion, vacuum your abs in and crunch them down into a tensed position.

The ab and thigh pose is one of the hardest to execute because it requires excellent flexibility in the pectoral girdle and shoulder joint. Yet this pose should be the one you rehearse most often. To improve, practice it when you do your lat and ab work.

Even if you're a noncompetitive bodybuilder, you should still follow this training/stretching/posing sequence. It will result in sharper muscularity and improved posture and carriage.

16 THE OPTIMUM REST INTERVAL

My recommended set sequence for each exercise is as follows: 1 warm-up set, 3 to 5 heavy pyramid sets (increasing the poundage each time and lowering the number of reps), and 1 to 2 high-rep sets (exhaustion sets). Put another way, you start off training a muscle slow and heavy, the way a powerlifter trains. You then finish training the muscle fast and intense, as a bodybuilder does.

Given these recommendations, how much rest should you take between each set in this sequence?

Between your warm-up set and first pyramid set, 30 seconds of rest will suffice. It's a different story for the pyramid sets, however. This is the part of the sequence in which you're building muscular density and thickness. You should pyramid up to the maximum weight you can lift by your last pyramid set. At that point, you may be down to just 1, 2, or 3 reps.

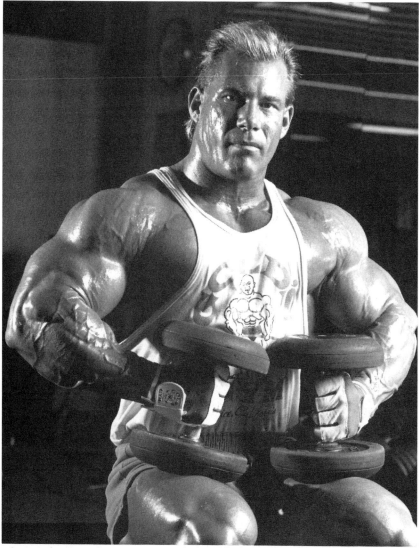

Massive Rick Stephenson begins a set of dumbbell curls. *Photo by Ralph DeHaan.*

Because of this level of heavy training, the amount of rest taken between pyramid sets becomes critical. Between these sets, I advise a rest interval of 2 to 5 minutes—the amount of time a powerlifter takes when training. This interval gives you ample time to repay your "oxygen debt." With short bursts of effort, oxygen can't be supplied fast enough for the recovery of the muscle. This debt is like a loan from the bank—borrowed money that has to be repaid. Your oxygen debt is paid back in installments as you catch your breath during the rest period between sets.

That way, you have enough oxygen to power your next heavy pyramid set. If you start another set while you're still breathless and your muscles haven't recovered, you may not be able to go as heavy as you want to. The muscles won't be worked to their full potential.

Shorten your rest between sets during your exhaustion sets. This is the portion of the workout sequence in which you're building cardiovascular density and endurance. Reducing the rest interval to 30 to 60 seconds enhances these fitness factors.

Keep in mind, too, that you should be stretching between all exercise sets. This takes up about 10 to 15 seconds of your rest interval and makes your workouts more productive.

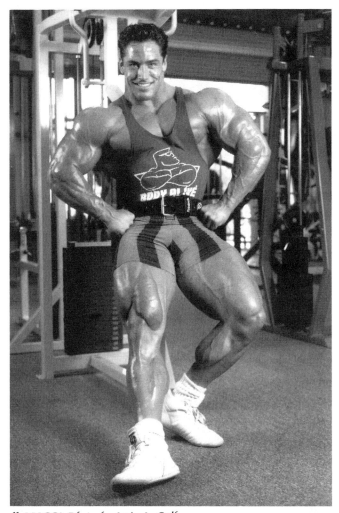

That's what you call MASS! *Photo by Irvin J. Gelb.*

17 SCULPTING THE OUTER SWEEP

The quadriceps muscles of the legs get subjected to some intense work. That's good. But sometimes you need to sharpen portions of the quads for better shape and definition. One area that demands attention is the vastus externus, better known as the "outer sweep." The largest of the four quadriceps muscles, the vastus externus forms the outside rim of the frontal thighs.

I find this part of the physique to be one of the most neglected on bodybuilders, even among the best-trained professionals. One reason has to do with the stance taken on squats and leg presses. In fact, I can tell by looking at a person's quads how he or she stands when performing these exercises.

The first step for improving your outer sweep is to fatigue your quads with squats—squats performed a special way to target and isolate the outer sweep. To begin, take a wide stance and angle your toes out. Descend slowly to a deep position—past the point at which your thighs are parallel to the floor. When descending, always sit back.

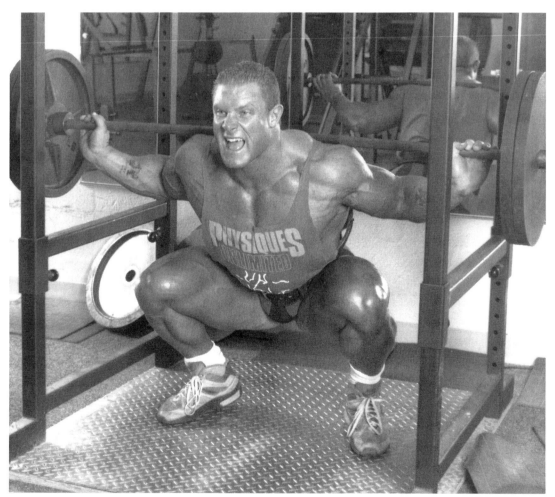

Press up from your heels to work the outer sweep, as John Caldarelli demonstrates. *Photo by Irvin J. Gelb.*

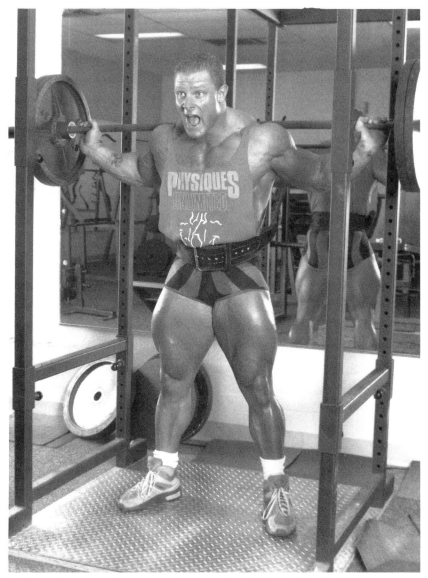

John Caldarelli performs an intense set of squats. *Photo by Irvin J. Gelb.*

The key to isolating the outer sweep is to push up from your heels on the ascent of the exercise. Curling your toes upward will help distribute your weight on your heels. As you come up, drive your hips forward and press your knees out. Upon rising, force your knees out and come up under the weight.

Perform 3 to 4 heavy sets of 8 to 12 reps each, pyramiding your poundages. Follow these with high-rep sets to exhaust the quads. Try to do 2 or more sets of 15 to 25 reps, using the technique explained above. Once you've finished your squats—your legs should feel a little shaky—move on to the leg press.

Place a two-inch-thick wooden board against the platform. With a medium stance, position your feet on the board. Bend your knees and lower the weight slowly, as deeply as you can. In fact, bring your knees just to your armpits. Now push back up with your heels. You should feel the stress on your outer thighs.

Aim for 3 to 4 heavy pyramid sets of leg presses. These should be followed by 2 to 3 high-rep exhaustion sets. When incorporating any heavy leg exercises like squats or leg presses in your routine, be sure to take in enough quality calories to support this level of training.

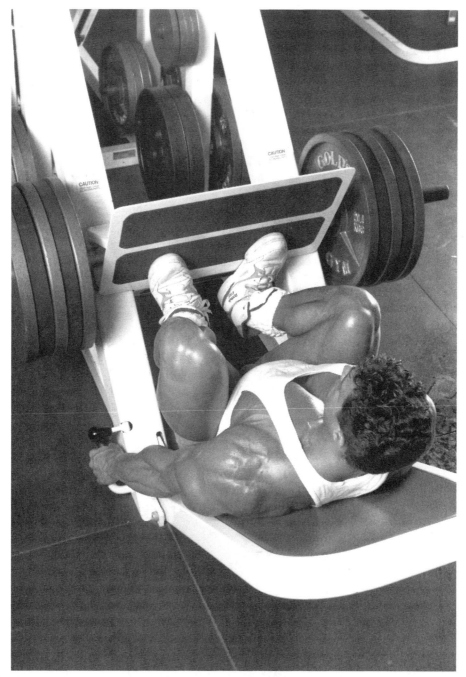

With the leg press, you can work various angles of your quads by altering your stance and the platform and changing the point from which you push. *Photo by Irvin J. Gelb.*

Another tip: Don't overlook hack squats as a way to sculpt the outer sweep. Although this exercise is considered a frontal quad movement, you can target your outer sweep, too. Simply widen your foot placement on the platform and angle your toes out slightly. Lower yourself to a deep position so that your thighs are parallel to the platform. Then push up from your heels. Return to the initial position. Keep your legs and glutes tight throughout the range of motion.

Include these techniques of training the outer thighs in your leg routine once a week. In several months, you should see a big difference.

OUTER SWEEP ROUTINE

Exercise	Sets and Reps
Squats (Curl toes upward and press up from heels.)	**Pyramid Sets** Warm-up set, 10 to 12 reps Set #1: 12 to 15 reps Set #2: 10 to 12 reps Set #3: 8 to 10 reps Set #4: 6 to 8 reps **Exhaustion Sets** Set #5: 15 to 25 reps Set #6: 15 to 25 reps
Leg press or hack squats (Press up from the heels.)	**Pyramid Sets** Warm-up set, 10 to 12 reps Set #1: 12 to 15 reps Set #2: 10 to 12 reps Set #3: 8 to 10 reps **Exhaustion Sets** Set #4: 15 to 25 reps Set #5: 15 to 25 reps

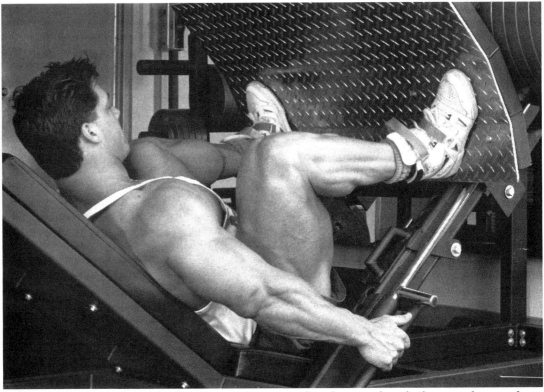

To isolate your quads on the leg press, place your feet low on the platform and press from the balls of your feet. *Photo by Irvin J. Gelb.*

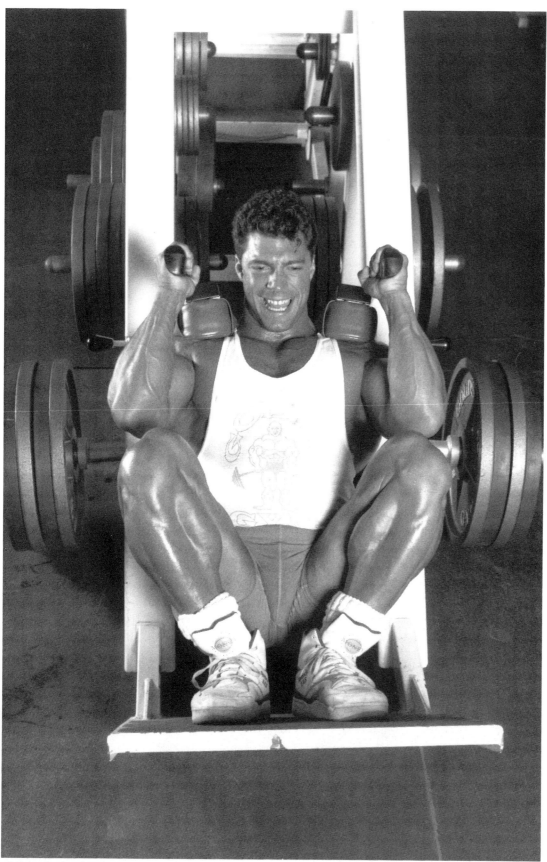

Although the hack squat is a frontal quad exercise, you can work your outer sweep by angling your feet out and pushing up from your heels. *Photo by Irvin J. Gelb.*

18 INNER THIGH DEFINITION

Chances are, you spend a lot of workout time on your quads and hamstrings. Most people do. Several other leg muscles deserve equal time: the adductors, a group of three muscles that makes up most of the inner thigh; the gracilis, a long, slender muscle on the outermost portion of the inner thigh; and the pectineus, located just below the groin. Together, these muscles assist in exercises involving the hips and quads. Keeping the inner thighs strong helps prevent injury during heavy leg work. By targeting this area, you can also firm up flabby thighs.

What's the best way to strengthen and develop the inner thighs? It's not necessarily with thigh adduction exercises using special machines or cables, although these offer some benefit, but with an exercise called the "power squat." It works not only the inner thighs but the hips as well. Here's how to do it:

- Instead of positioning the barbell across your shoulders as you would with a regular squat, place it at a lower point on your back. The bar should fit in a groove formed by your shoulder blades. Keep your elbows pressed back and up to prevent the bar from sliding down your back.
- Take a wide stance and curl your toes upward to keep your weight on your heels.
- Descend slowly to a deep position. Sit back as you lower and push your rear end back slightly.
- As you press out of the bottom position, force your knees out. Then come up under the weight. Drive your hips forward on the ascent. This exercise makes your inner thighs and hips feel like they were worked hard.

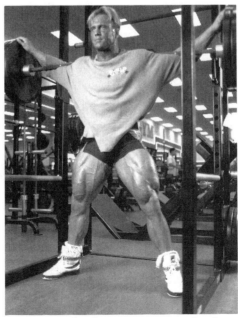

With the power squat, you position the bar across your back rather than your shoulders. *Photo by Irvin J. Gelb.*

19 TARGET SQUATTING FOR THE FRONTAL THIGH

There are many different styles of squatting, each with its own purpose and function. Conventional squats, for example, hit the entire lower body—the glutes, quads, and hamstrings—while others target specific muscle groups of the lower body. One of the most effective "specialty" squats is the high-bar squat, used to target the quads of the frontal thigh. With this exercise, less emphasis is placed on the glutes and hamstrings.

The high-bar squat is usually performed with your heels elevated on a board. The elevation lets you press upward from the balls of your feet, a motion that directly isolates the quads.

To begin, place your feet about twelve inches apart. This is a more narrow stance than you would take when performing a conventional squat. Your toes should point forward.

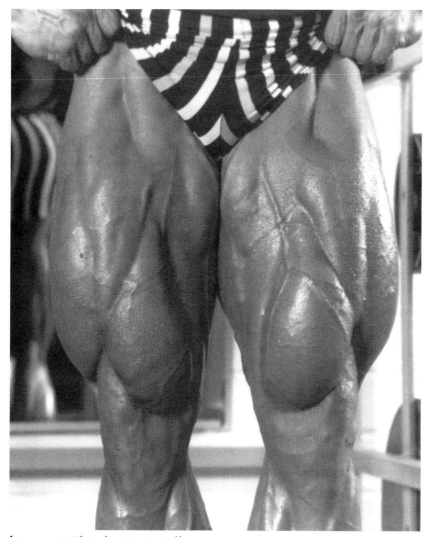

Incredible leg mass! *Photo by Irvin J. Gelb.*

Descend slowly to a deep position, directing your knees forward and over your toes. Then press back up, using the balls of your feet. Be sure to push your hips forward and straighten your back as you return to the initial position.

The best-known squat for the frontal thighs is the hack squat, described in section #17. To keep the emphasis on the front quads, place your feet close together on the platform. Point your toes forward. Lower yourself as deeply as possible and stay tight throughout the exercise. Press up from the balls of your feet.

If you feel that your frontal thighs need extra work, I suggest that you include the high-bar squat and hack squats in your leg routine. Here's a routine that will help you sharpen your frontal thighs:

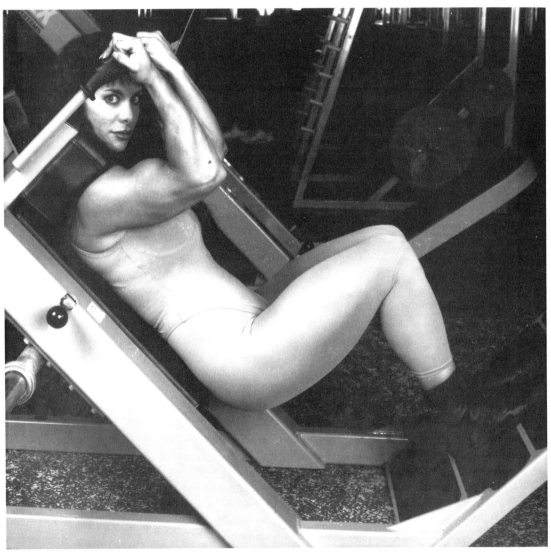

Athena uses hack squats in her leg routine. *Photo by Jimmie D. King.*

FRONTAL THIGH ROUTINE

Exercise	Sets & Reps
High-bar squat (Pyramid up in poundages.)	Warm-up set (unloaded bar) 10 reps Set #2: 8 to 12 reps Set #3: 8 to 12 reps Set #4: 8 to 12 reps Set #5: 8 to 12 reps
Hack squat (Take a narrow stance and press with the balls of your feet. Pyramid your poundages.)	Set #1: 12 to 15 reps Set #2: 8 to 12 reps Set #3: 8 to 12 reps Set #4: 8 to 12 reps
Leg extensions (See section #20 for some tips on exercise performance.)	Perform 2 to 4 sets of 15 to 25 reps

20 A MORE EFFECTIVE LEG EXTENSION

The leg extension is often called a "finishing exercise" because it helps carve out the separations among the four muscles that make up the quadriceps muscles of the frontal thigh. What's more, many bodybuilders like to use the exercise at the start of their leg routine as a warm-up for the quadriceps. A major advantage of the leg extension is that it lets you contract the quads more fully than you can with other leg exercises, and this stimulates the muscle fibers more deeply.

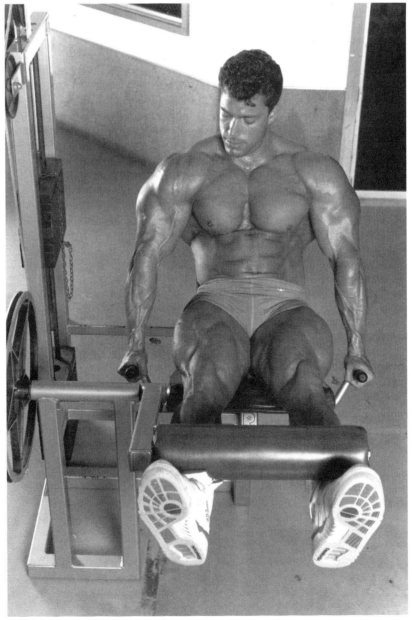

At the top of the leg extension, try to lift your knees and lower quads off the bench, as Bob Cicherillo demonstrates. *Photo by Irvin J. Gelb.*

There are two key points of execution when performing the leg extensions. First, make sure you achieve full lock-out at the top of the exercise to get maximum stimulation. With the insteps of your feet hooked under the padded roller, lift upward in an arc. When your knee joints are fully extended, contract your quads as hard as you can to lock out. Hold your quads in the contracted position for a half second. Second, try to lift your lower quads and knees off the bench. Squeeze your quads hard as you lift.

The leg extension is a finishing exercise in another regard. It's an excellent way to end your quadriceps routine. After performing squats and leg presses, for example, finish off with 4 high-rep (exhaustion) sets of leg extensions—15 to 25 reps each set. Exhaustion sets help build cardiovascular density and endurance, as well as muscular separation, in the quads. For better results, rep out to muscular failure on every exhaustion set.

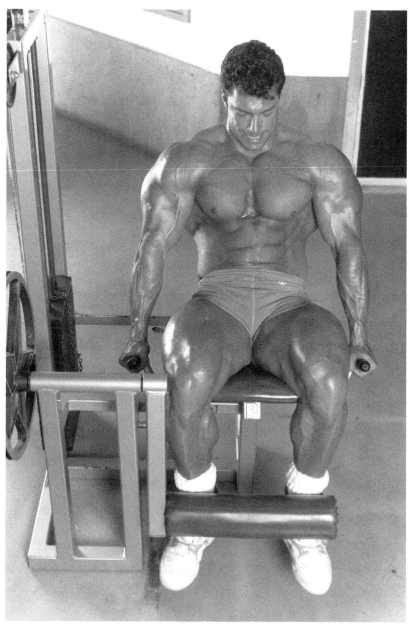

On leg extensions, lower the weight using the strength of your opposing muscles. *Photo by Irvin J. Gelb.*

21 THE PERFECT LEG EXERCISE

There's no question that squats are among the best exercises for building quadriceps. The exercise has some limiting factors, however. It can be stressful on the lower back and knees if performed incorrectly. It can overbuild the glutes and spread the hips. And it requires tremendous lower back strength. Once you surpass 20 reps with squats, your quads may give out, causing your lower back muscles to take over. If these muscles are weak, the risk of back injury is increased.

A type of squat that overcomes these limitations is the belt squat. It uses a special squatting apparatus featuring a rectangular platform with an open area in the center. An attached pole with a sliding handle is positioned front and center of this platform and is used to guide your vertical path while squatting. You wear a weight belt harness attached to plates.

The belt squat gives you a superb training edge for building not only the quads but other systems of the body. Here's what I mean:

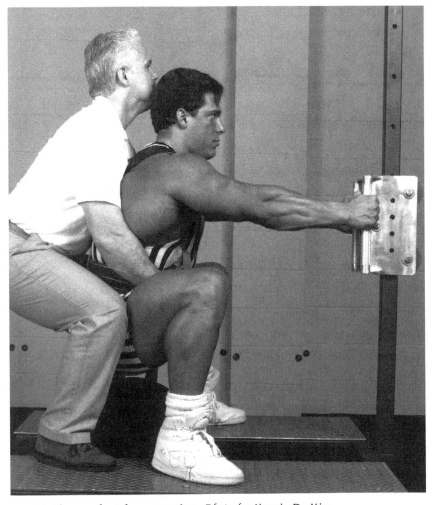

The belt squat is the perfect leg exercise. *Photo by Jimmie D. King.*

Lower Back Protection. With regular squats, the goal is to go as heavy as you can, usually in a pyramid sequence. But the heavier the weight is, the more you tend to sacrifice form. When squats start feeling hard, for example, a lot of bodybuilders begin using their legs *less* in the exercise. The glutes go up and back instead of forward. This action shifts the stress directly to the lower back, placing undue strain there.

The design of most belt squat machines dictates proper form. To begin with, you automatically maintain an upright position throughout the exercise. No leverage is placed on your lower back either. In addition, all the poundage is concentrated on your legs, not on your back. The entire training load is concentrated on the muscles of the legs and glutes, forcing you to work your legs *hard*. And that translates into greater gains.

Increased Golgi Tendon Reflex (GTR) Threshold. One way to increase your GTR threshold is to train with high reps and heavy weights. You could try squats for this, but it's difficult to do high-rep squats with heavy poundages.

This isn't the case with the belt squat machine, because the total load is on the legs. In fact, you can do many times the number of repetitions on the belt squat as you can with regular squats. I like to employ spotted reps with the belt squat so you can give the exercise all-out effort, using 100 to 200 pounds more than you can safely lift on your own. The spotter helps center your weight and keeps your momentum going for maximum intensity. Each time you train on the belt squat with a spotter, you're able to do more and more reps, with higher poundages.

With the belt squat—unlike regular squats—you can train with heavy weights and high repetitions, as well as with forced reps. Heavy weights increase the GTR threshold, and high repetitions develop greater cardiovascular fitness and overall stamina.

In addition, high-rep training leads to better neural control of your muscles by opening up "high-threshold" nerve paths in the muscle fibers. These take more energy to activate. High reps lower the threshold, allowing a greater number of muscle fibers to fire. More muscle comes into play as a result, and strength and mass are increased. I once worked with a powerlifter who lifted competitively in the 220-pound weight class. He could never seem to break the 600-pound mark on his squat. After just four months of training on the belt squat, he increased his competition squat to 740 pounds. With the belt squat, you can find out what your strength barriers are and then train well past them.

Quad Shaping. On the belt squat, you can take advantage of the total focused overload placed on the legs in another way—to shape portions of the quads like the outer sweep. To build the outer sweep, angle your toes outward and press up from your heels on each rep.

Fat-Burning Capacity. High-rep, heavy-poundage training like that performed on the belt squat can boost your fat-burning capacity by altering the characteristics of your muscle fibers. This type of high-volume training actually changes pure fast-twitch muscle fibers (the kind that fatigue quickly and burn glycogen for energy) into fast-twitch oxidative muscle fibers, which burn fat. (See section #12.) High-volume training increases the number of mitochondria in the muscle cells. With more mitochondria in muscle cells, the fast-twitch muscle fibers burn more fat. Through the high-volume training on the belt squat, your body becomes a fat-burning machine.

Safe Exercise Performance. For extra safety on the belt squat, I recommend that you use a spotter on every set. To begin the exercise, stand erect and grasp the handle in front of you. Stand with your toes slightly outward. Keep your weight centered. Have your spotter stand closely behind you with his arms around your waist holding the front of the weight belt. Lower to a position below parallel. Push your knees out and press your hips forward. Return to the initial position and lock your knees hard. Even if you and your spotter can't finish a rep, the exercise is still very safe because you can sit down on the plates.

The Ultimate Leg Routine. Here is the belt squat routine I recommend for developing strength, power, and musculature. Many famous bodybuilders have used this routine (and lived to tell about it!). It has earned quite a reputation over the years because of its grueling intensity. A note of caution: This is an advanced routine designed for well-trained bodybuilders on high-calorie, nutrient-dense nutrition programs. On the last set, you must rotate new spotters every 20 reps.

BELT SQUAT ROUTINE

Sets	Poundage	Reps
Set #1, Warm-up, spotted	100	20
Set #2, Warm-up, spotted	200	15
Set #3, Warm-up, spotted	300	10
Set #4, Heavy, spotted	400	Maximum
Set #5, High-rep, spotted	100 to 200	40 to 100

---

22 TIGHTER GLUTES

Most women know that lower body fat—that type that accumulates around the thighs and glutes—is stubborn to shed when compared to other parts of the body, particularly the abs. As frustrating as it is, this stubbornness is a necessary design of Nature. Lower body fat cells serve as a reservoir of energy in anticipation of pregnancy and lactation. In fact, the only time lower body fat is easily released is during lactation, when more fat is required for energy.

Although you can't "spot-reduce" lower body fat, you can firm up this area by performing specific exercises that isolate the major muscles of the hip, the gluteus maximus, the gluteus medius, and the gluteus minimus. Isolation exercises will do more than anything else to tighten these muscles and give them a firmer, rounder appearance.

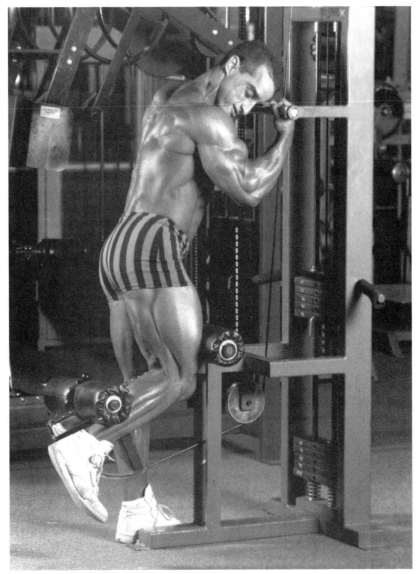

Matt McLaughlin works out on the standing leg curl machine. *Photo by Irvin J. Gelb.*

Additionally, large storage depots of fat, regardless of where they are on the body, typically have poor circulation, making metabolism of fat very difficult and causing "cellulite." Cellulite is a type of fat on the thighs, hips, and buttocks that gives a dimpled appearance to the skin. By exercising these areas, the muscles contract, and more blood moves into the area. Circulation is improved, and the metabolism of fat is optimized.

By working your glutes hard two or three times a week, you should see results within two months. In addition, be sure to follow a low-fat, high-calorie nutrition eating plan and a consistent program of daily aerobics. Both will maximize fat-burning.

Now, get to the gym and "burn your buns" with the following routine:

Exercise #1: Glute Squats. Take a stance slightly wider than shoulder width. Descend slowly—past the point at which your thighs are parallel to the floor—while keeping your weight on your heels. Sit back as you move through the exercise. This action keeps the leverage and emphasis off the frontal thigh and squarely on the glutes. Slowly return to the starting position. Keep your glutes tight throughout the exercise. At the top of the exercise push your hips forward, lock your knees, and squeeze your glutes hard. Perform 3 to 5 sets of glute squats, increasing the poundage each time, for 8 to 12 reps.

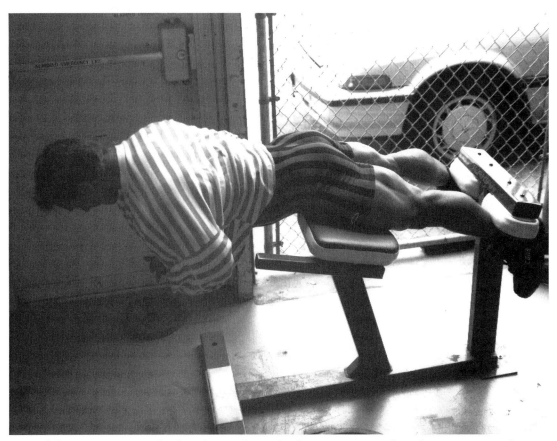

By stabilizing your torso farther forward on the hyperextension bench, you can work your glute/hamstring tie-in. *Photo by Irvin J. Gelb.*

Exercise #2: Reverse Hyperextensions. Immediately follow the glute squat exercise with reverse hyperextensions, without resting between exercises. Lie facedown on the hyperextension bench so that your legs extend off the bench and form a right angle to your torso. Keeping your glutes tight and your legs together, lift your legs upward in an arc. Squeeze your glutes even more tightly as you reach the contracted position. At this point, push your heels back and lock your knees in a half-swing, half-kick motion. Squeeze your glutes hard again. Perform between 20 and 50 repetitions.

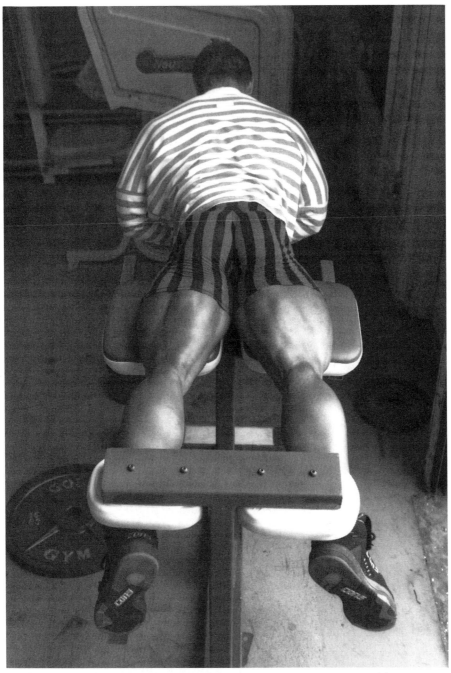

When using the hyperextension as a glute/hamstring exercise, raise and lower your torso using the strength of your hamstrings. *Photo by Irvin J. Gelb.*

Exercise #3: Leg Press with Glute Emphasis. To work the glutes on the leg press, place your feet high on the platform and curl your toes upward. With your heels, push the platform up and down in a single continuous movement. Keep constant tension on all working muscles as you push through the exercise.

Perform 3 to 5 sets of leg presses, increasing the poundage each time, for 8 to 12 reps.

Exercise #4: Straight-Leg Deadlift. This exercise is a pure glute and hamstring isolation movement if done correctly. Pick up the barbell (dumbbells can be used, too) and begin the exercise from the upright position. As you start the exercise, arch your back and push your abs toward the floor. Pivot at the hip joint, not the lower back. The first pull should be with your hamstrings. As you continue to lift the weight, tighten your glutes, lock your knees, and push your hips forward. Squeeze your glutes hard at the top. Keep everything tight as you perform the exercise. Do 3 to 5 sets of straight-leg deadlifts, for 8 to 12 reps. Finish off your glute routine with one more set of reverse hyperextensions, performing between 20 and 50 reps.

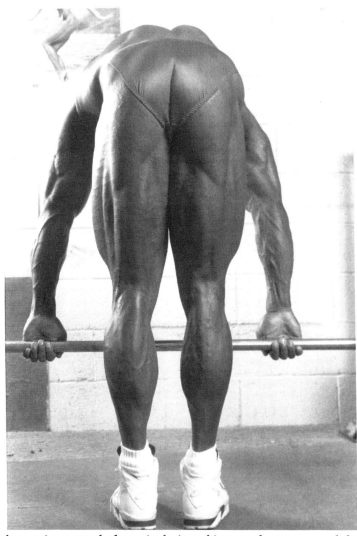

Well-separated hamstrings result from isolating this muscle group and focusing on strict form during exercise. *Photo by Irvin J. Gelb.*

23 BALANCED HAMSTRING DEVELOPMENT

It's easy to fall into the trap of undertraining the hamstrings. Being on the posterior of the physique, they're not as visible as the quadriceps and are often worked less intensely as a result. Overdeveloping the quads at the expense of the hamstrings is a problem not only of appearance but also of muscular balance. Where there is an imbalance in the ratio of quadriceps to hamstring strength, the risk of muscle tears or pulls is increased.

These problems can be avoided with proper exercise selection and good exercise form. The leg curl, for example, is one of the most effective exercises for the hamstrings, and there's a way you can make it even better. When performing this exercise, keep your hips pressed into the pad. Lift your knees up off the pad at the top of the exercise. This subtle movement really "burns" the hamstrings.

The bent-knee straight-leg deadlift is a variation on the straight-leg version. The difference is that on the bent-knee deadlift, you keep your knees slightly bent rather than stiff. This slight change in position isolates the glute/hamstring tie-in (the point at the top of the legs where these two muscles meet), making the exercise the best movement for this area.

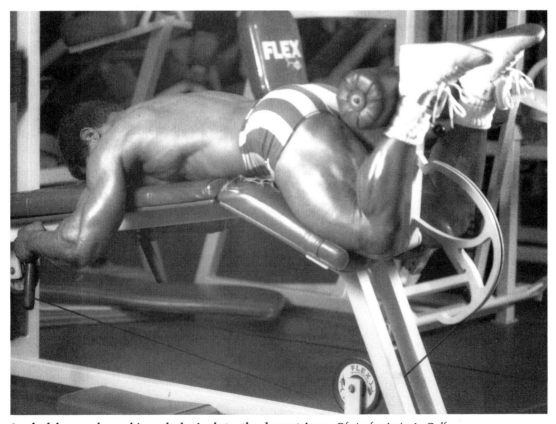

Angled leg curl machines help isolate the hamstrings. *Photo by Irvin J. Gelb.*

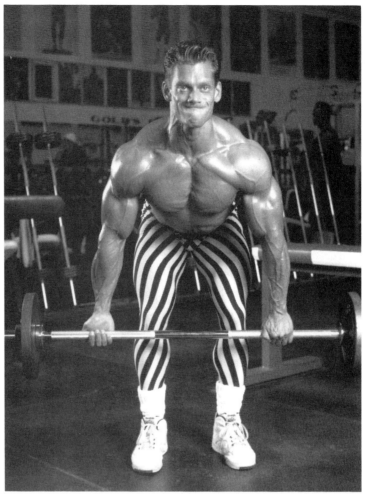

Partial straight-leg deadlifts help you develop the glute/hamstring tie-in. *Photo by Irvin J. Gelb.*

The shape of the glute/hamstring tie-in says a lot about how hard you train and how conscientious you are about fine-tuning your physique. Bent-knee straight-leg deadlifts will give you that tight, well-defined look at the tie-in point.

This exercise must be executed with full attention to form. Pick up the barbell or dumbbells and begin the exercise in the upright position. Bend your knees slightly, arch your back, and extend your glutes out. Maintain this position while lowering the bar slowly. Don't lower the bar all the way to the floor, just to a point under your knees or wherever you feel a deep stretch in your hamstrings. At this point, stretch hard, keeping your lower back arched. As you pull the bar back up, push your hips forward, lock your knees, and contract your glutes hard.

Hyperextensions are another excellent exercise for the glute/hamstring tie-in. Most people think of this exercise as a back movement—and it is. But if you stabilize your torso farther forward on the hyperextension bench, you bring your glutes and hamstrings into play instead of your back.

To begin, position yourself on the bench so that your torso is free to pivot at the hip joint. With your hands behind your head, lower your torso to the floor while keeping your upper back arched. Then slowly lift back up until your upper body is at a point just higher than parallel to the floor.

HAMSTRING ROUTINE	
Exercise	**Sets & Reps**
Bent-knee straight-leg deadlift (Pyramid up in poundages.)	Set #1: 12 to 15 reps Set #2: 12 to 15 reps Set #3: 12 to 15 reps Set #4: 12 to 15 reps
Leg curls (Pyramid up in poundages.)	Set #1: 10 to 12 reps Set #2: 10 to 12 reps Set #3: 10 to 12 reps Set #4: 15 to 25 reps (Lower poundages for exhaustion sets.) Set #5: 25 to 30 reps (Lower poundages for exhaustion sets.)
Hyperextension (Position torso forward on the bench for greater glute action.)	Aim for a maximum number of reps.

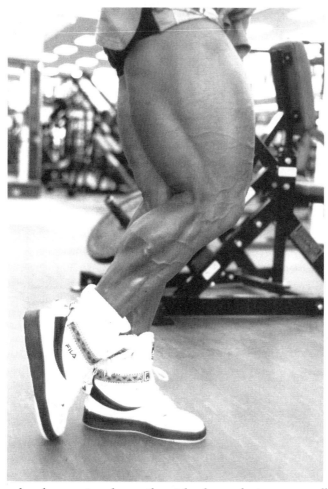

Balanced hamstring development reduces the risk of muscle tears or pulls and gives a proportional look to the leg. *Photo by Irvin J. Gelb.*

24 CALF TRAINING TRICKS FOR THE GASTROCNEMIUS

The gastrocnemius is the largest and most visible muscle of the lower leg. It has two heads—an inner head (the larger of the two) and an outer head. On most physiques, the outer head lags in development and requires extra work to bring it up to potential. A special technique performed on standing calf raises will do the trick.

Place your feet on the standing calf raise platform. As you raise up, cock your heels outward just slightly. Then shift all of your weight onto your big toes and press up. Lock your knees out hard at the top. You should feel the isolation

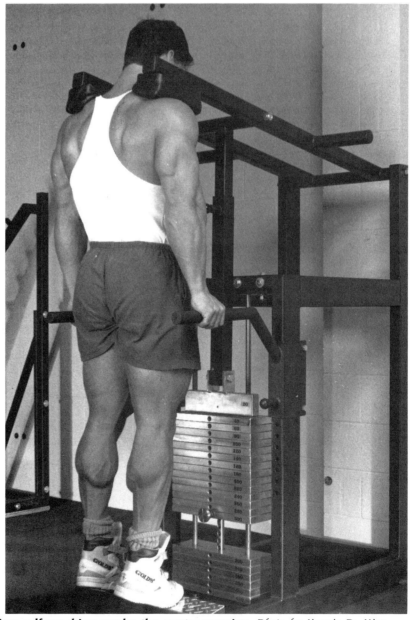

The standing calf machine works the gastrocnemius. *Photo by Jimmie D. King.*

on your outer head. Lower slowly to get a deep stretch at the bottom of the exercise.

Be careful not to assume a pigeon-toed stance as you cock your heels out. Although it changes the angle of the foot, a pigeon-toed stance doesn't necessarily work the outer head. Isolating the outer head still depends on distributing your weight on your big toe and pressing up from there.

You can apply similar techniques to the inner head, also using the standing calf machine. This time cock your heels inward slightly and press up from the outer portion of your feet. Lock your knees at the top. You should feel the emphasis on your inner head.

These techniques for the outer and inner heads are effective if you need to "play catch-up" in building shape and size in your calf muscles.

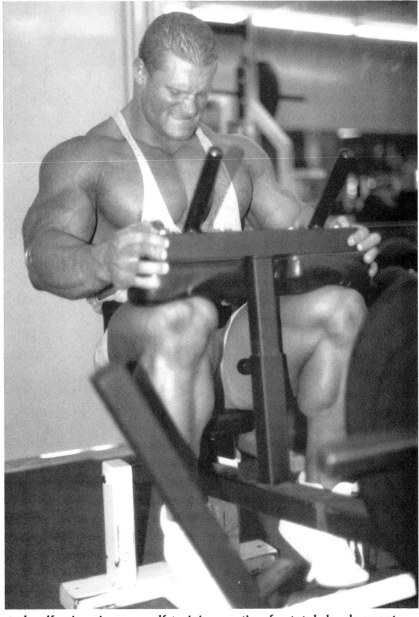

Include seated calf raises in your calf training routine for total development.
Photo by Irvin J. Gelb.

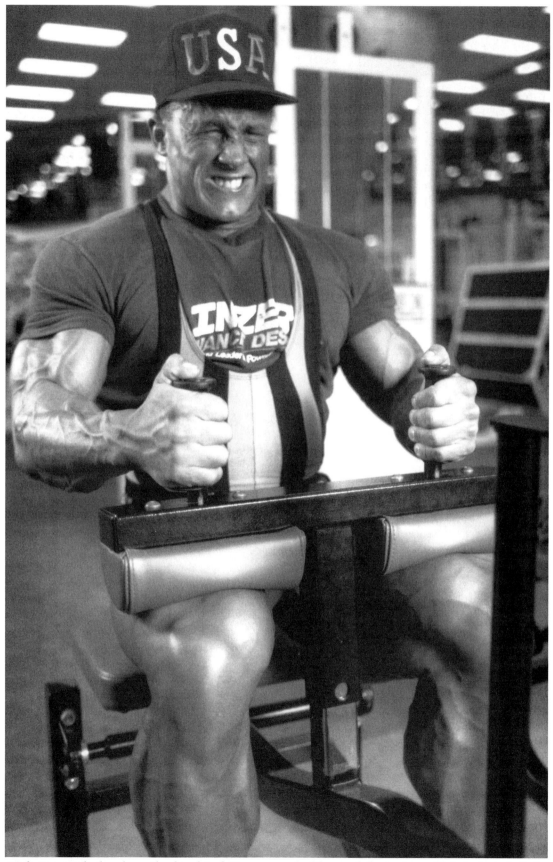

High-rep work develops the hard-to-fatigue muscle fibers of the calves. *Photo by Irvin J. Gelb.*

25 A HIGH-VOLUME SOLEUS WORKOUT

The soleus is a broad, flat muscle located underneath the gastrocnemius. The best exercise for working the soleus is the seated calf raise. How you position yourself in the seated calf machine, however, makes a big difference in how the calf muscles are worked. For example, most people sit in the machine with their legs in a 90-degree angle—a position that brings too much of the gastrocnemius into play. To work the soleus, you must break that angle by moving your legs farther back in the machine toward your body. In other words, your lower legs should be almost directly underneath you.

The soleus is composed mostly of slow-twitch muscle fibers, which can keep contracting for long periods of time, without fatiguing. In terms of growth, these fibers respond best to high-intensity, high-repetition training, including forced repetitions. Here is a routine designed to work the soleus to the max. You'll know you're doing it intensely enough if it hurts!

Exercise #1: Seated Calf Raises. Sit in the machine with your knees under the padded bar. Be sure to break the 90-degree angle as explained above. On each rep, lift your feet up as high as possible, then lower deeply for a good stretch. Perform 2 to 4 sets of these with 50 to 100 reps each time.

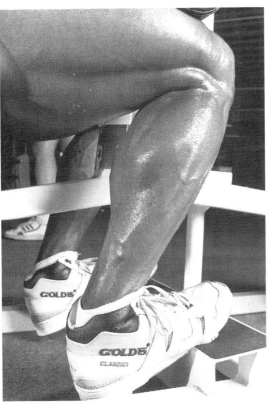

On seated calf raises, break the 90-degree angle with your calves to better isolate the soleus. *Photo by Ralph DeHaan.*

Exercise #2: Calf Squats. Perform these between each set of calf exercises. This exercise is the only way you can totally contract both the gastrocnemius and the soleus at the same time. To begin, position the balls of your feet on a block of wood or on the foot platform of the standing calf machine. Grasp the equipment with both hands. Squat down and keep your heels under your glutes, with your feet and knees pressed together. Raise up as high as you can on the balls of your feet. At the top, press your glutes to your heels. Then lower to a deep stretch. Continue raising and lowering in this fashion for about 20 to 30 reps.

Exercise #3: Toe Presses. Depending on how this exercise is performed, you can isolate either the soleus or the gastrocnemius. Position yourself in the incline leg press machine with the balls of your feet on the lower edge of the foot platform. To work the soleus, keep your knees slightly bent; to work the gastrocnemius, keep your knees locked. With your legs in position, press back and forth with your feet, getting a good stretch in each direction. Attempt as many sets and reps as you can. Make sure to perform calf squats between each set of toe presses.

The best approach for working the calf muscles is to train them two days in a row, followed by a day of rest. In your first workout, emphasize soleus work; in the next workout, emphasize gastrocnemius work.

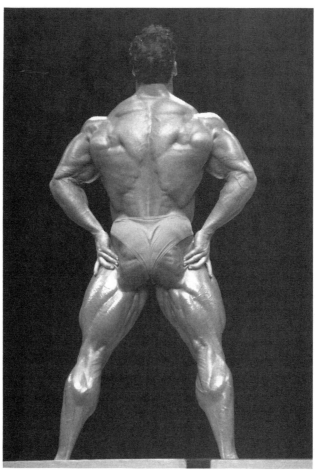

Diamond-shaped calves. *Photo by Irvin J. Gelb.*

26 PECTORAL POWER

Who doesn't want broad, muscular pecs? There are two ways to get them—even if genetics are not in your favor. Before I explain how, let's consider some important points about pectoral anatomy.

Most people don't realize that the chest is actually composed of three muscles: the pectoralis major, which covers the entire chest; the pectoralis minor, a thin, flat, triangular muscle that arises from the third, fourth, and fifth ribs; and the subclavius. The subclavius is a small triangular muscle located between the clavicle and the first rib at the top of the chest. The fleshy fibers of the subclavius angle up and out, inserting into a deep groove under the surface of the clavicle.

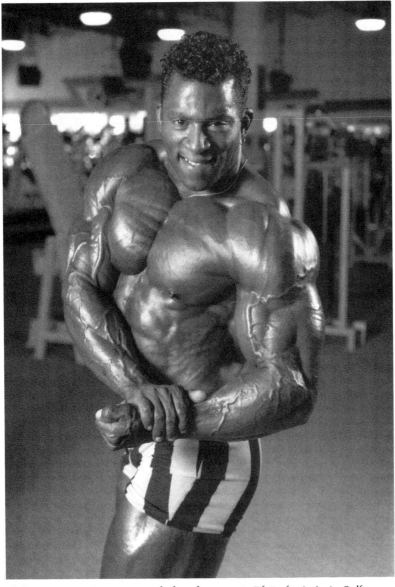

Darryl Stafford has impressive pectoral development. *Photo by Irvin J. Gelb.*

For complete development of all three muscles, you must find a way to place the mechanical advantage on the upper portions of the pectoralis major. One way to achieve this is by using proper form when bench pressing. Most bodybuilders, however, rely too heavily on the strength of their front deltoids to push through the exercise. They drop their chest at the top of the exercise and then push up with their delts. The result is great front delts but flat, underdeveloped pectorals, especially in the upper region of the chest.

Your pectoral muscles can become thicker and fuller in a matter of weeks when you make certain adjustments in the way you perform bench presses. In fact, some people have felt a difference the first time they try my bench press technique. Here's how it works:

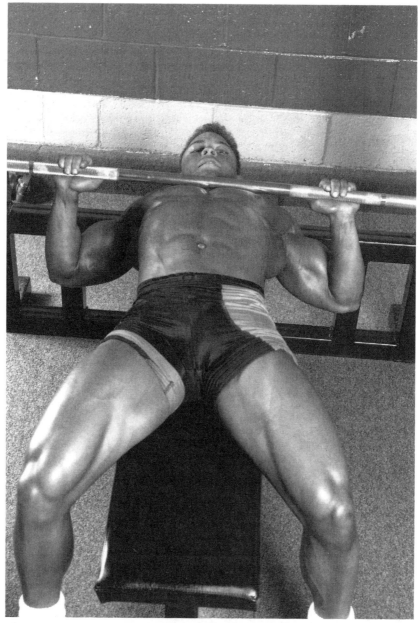

On the bench press, set up your pectoral girdle properly by pushing your shoulders down toward your waist and into the bench, as Kelly Pettiford demonstrates. *Photo by Irvin J. Gelb.*

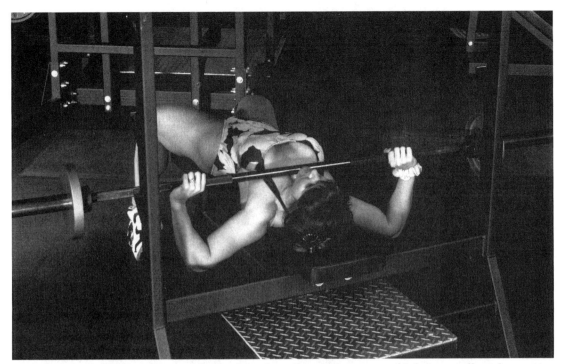

A variation of the bench press is the bench-to-the-neck press, which is excellent for upper pectoral development. As you lower the bar, pinch your chin to your chest. Then bring the bar down to this pinch point. *Photo by Jimmie D. King.*

Lie back on the bench and take a grip that is slightly wider than the width of your shoulders. Push your shoulders down toward your waist and back into the bench. They should feel as though they are under your body. This position sets up your pectoral girdle properly so that the mechanical advantage of the bench press is placed directly on the pectorals, rather than on the deltoids. Maintain this position throughout each set.

Next, push your chest forward and begin the exercise. At the top of the exercise, lock your elbows out while arching your sternum and pressing it up. Unless you lock out in this fashion, you won't work your upper pecs. Squeeze your shoulders down toward your lower lats and pec minor.

In addition to using correct bench press form, you can maximize your chest development in another way: bench pressing on an arched incline bench. This bench is constructed so that the part supporting your back is curved in an arc. On this type of equipment, it's nearly impossible to bench incorrectly or to misplace leverage on the delts and lower pecs. The bench positions your body so that your chest is arched up, your head is tilted back, and your rear end is down. This position forces the mechanical advantage squarely on your upper pecs, completely isolates your upper pecs, and improves muscular stimulation.

And because less stress and pressure are placed on the shoulders, the likelihood of injury is reduced. Benching on an arched incline is safer and more productive than on a regular flat bench.

By combining proper bench press form with the right equipment, you can have unprecedented pectoral gains and break genetic barriers to achieve maximum chest development.

27 CHISELING THE INNER PECS

For sharper inner pec development, try this variation of the dumbbell fly exercise. Lie on the bench, setting up your pectoral girdle in the same position used in the bench press. Work your shoulders under your body and keep them pressed down and into the bench. Begin your set by arching your back.

With palms pointing inward, extend your arms to a position directly over your head. Bend your arms slightly and lower them out to the sides as low as possible to get a good stretch. Slowly return the weights to the starting position. At the top of the movement, try to touch your elbows together, not the dumbbells. This action isolates the inner pecs and adds muscular detail to this area.

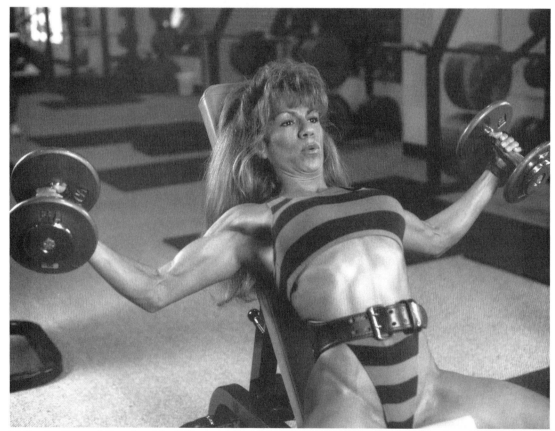

At the bottom of the dumbbell fly exercise, be sure to get a good stretch. *Photo by Irvin J. Gelb.*

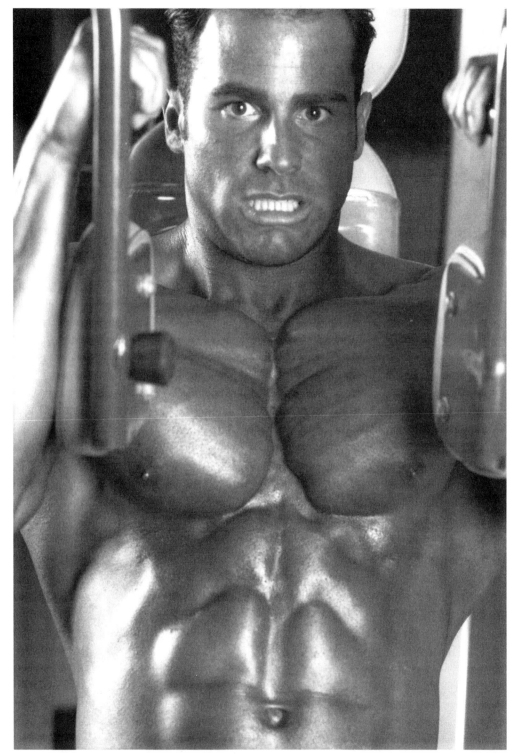

When performing machine presses, squeeze your pecs at the top of the exercise to thoroughly work the muscle. *Photo by Irvin J. Gelb.*

28 A DEFINITION ROUTINE FOR THE PECS

A definition-producing exercise for the pecs is the cable crossover. It lets you work various sections of the pecs from different angles by simply adjusting the position of the pulleys. (The cable crossover can be performed on a flat, incline, or decline bench for even more versatility.) Here's what I mean:

In each of these variations, there's a trick you can apply to work more of the muscle. Start the exercise and bring your arms forward in the fly motion. It's here that most people stop and return to the initial position. But there's more you can do. At this point—the top of the exercise—try to bring your elbows together. Push your chest out as you would on a pressing movement and press your shoulders down. Then flex your lats and contract your chest hard. By starting the exercise like a dumbbell fly and finishing it like a bench press, you subject your pectoral muscles to additional work on each rep.

What follows is a pec routine using the cable crossover machine. Try it if you want to bring out more definition and striations in your pecs.

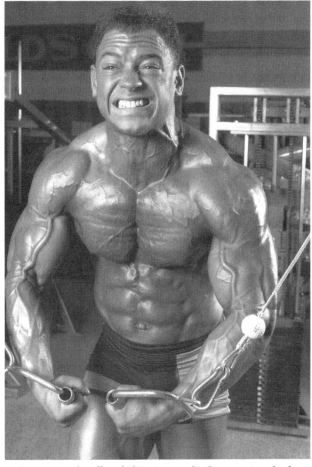

The cable crossover gives you the flexibility to work the pectorals from many different angles. *Photo by Irvin J. Gelb.*

Pulley Position	Angle	Section
Low	Cross pulleys in front of your face.	Upper pecs
High	Cross pulleys in front of your abs.	Middle and lower pecs
Middle*	Cross pulleys in front of your chest.	Entire pec area
Low, middle, or high	Step forward from the machine and reach behind your body as you pull forward.	Middle and outer pecs

* Machines such as the Parrillo Hardcore Advantage Cable Crossover Machine have the midposition capability; others do not.

CABLE CROSSOVER ROUTINE FOR THE PECS

Technique	Exercise	Sets & Reps
Superset #1: Follow each set of cable crossovers immediately with bench presses. Rest, then repeat the superset 3 more times.	Cable crossover (Set pulley in the low or middle position.)	4 sets of 10 to 15 reps
	Flat bench press	4 sets of 10 to 15 reps
Superset #2: Follow each set of incline dumbbell presses immediately with incline cable crossovers. Rest, then repeat the superset 3 more times.	Incline dumbbell press	3 sets of 8 to 12 reps
	Incline cable crossover (Set pulley at low position.)	3 sets of 10 to 15 reps
Superset #3: Follow each set of decline dumbbell bench presses immediately with cable crossovers. Rest, then repeat the superset 3 more times.	Decline dumbbell bench presses	3 sets of 8 to 12 reps
	Cable crossover (Set pulley in the high position.)	3 sets of 10 to 15 reps

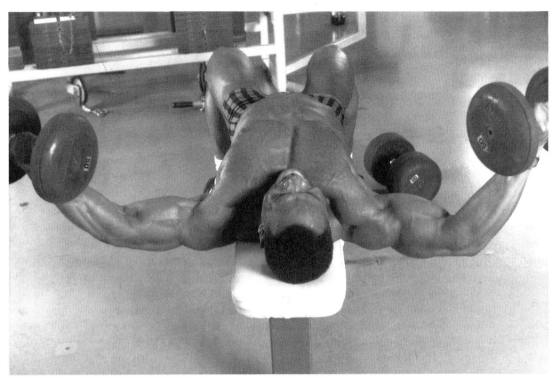

With dumbbell flies, it's important to keep your shoulders pressed into the bench throughout the exercise, as Derrick Whitsett shows. *Photo by Irvin J. Gelb.*

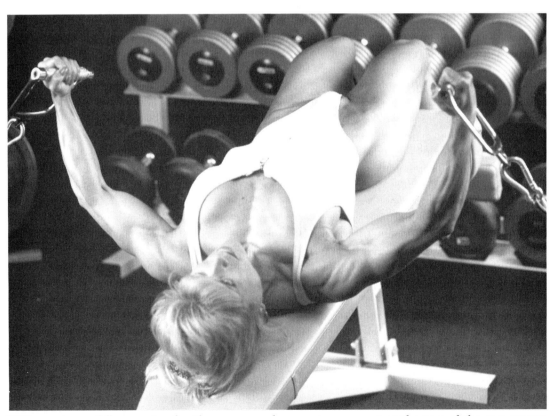

With any type of fly exercise for the pecs, push your sternum out at the top of the movement for better isolation of the chest. *Photo by Ralph DeHaan.*

29 ABSOLUTELY PERFECT ABS

Tight, well-muscled abs are a prized physique trait—one that's easy to achieve with the proper diet and the right exercise routine. Great abs lead not only to a great body but also to better health. In fact, mounting research shows that fat around the waist is a serious risk factor for heart disease, diabetes, high blood pressure, and high cholesterol. In women, abdominal fat may even raise the risk of breast and reproductive cancers.

As you put on fat, your body tends to distribute it in a certain order. In women, fat is parceled out first to the hips, buttocks, and thighs, then around the waist (just below the skin), and finally, within the abdominal cavity. Men, on the other hand, typically gain and store weight in the reverse order, accumulating more fat in the abdominal area. This pattern of abdominal fat distribution is not limited to men, nor is lower body fat distribution restricted to women. Both sexes, however, expand at the waist with age.

Many factors contribute to abdominal weight gain, including genetics and hormones, but perhaps the biggest offender is behavior. Overindulging on fatty foods, for example, leads to greater abdominal fat.

Dietary fat finds its way into fat cells with the help of enzymes. When you consume too much fat, enzymes split the fat into smaller components that can move into fat tissue for storage. Similarly, enzymes are responsible for mobilizing fat out of storage sites when it is needed for energy.

Another factor in abdominally distributed fat is "weight cycling"—repeated bouts of weight loss and weight gain, also known as "yo-yo" dieting. Research shows that people who go on and off low-calorie diets tend to gain more fat in the abdominal area, probably because weight cycling suppresses the metabolism, making it easier for the body to store fat. Another explanation is that weight cycling increases fat consumption. Once off your diet, you tend to eat more fatty foods. And that fat goes to the waistline.

It should encourage you to know that abdominal fat is easy to shed—much easier than lower body fat, which clings stubbornly to storage sites. This is because the enzymes in fat tissue of the abdominal region are very active, and there is a higher turnover of fat, particularly in response to low-fat dieting and exercise. In fact, enzyme action is even greater during exercise due to the release of adrenaline in response to activity. Adrenaline liberates fatty acids into the bloodstream so that the body can use them for fuel. Furthermore, abdominal fat seems highly sensitive to adrenaline. Compared to fat in other places, abdominal fat is more easily released.

The first step toward tight, "washboard" abs is a low-fat, nutrient-dense diet—one that's abundant in lean protein, starchy carbohydrates, and high-fiber vegetables.

Get to know the grams of dietary fat for each food in your diet by referring to a guide such as the U.S. Agriculture Department's *Composition of Foods Handbook* No. 8. You'll see that even though all your food choices are relatively low in fat, some foods have even fewer grams of fat per serving than others. For example, if you want to further lower your fat intake, try eating more fish and egg whites, since they are among the lowest in fat of all proteins. Be sure to avoid red meat and processed foods, which are loaded with fat. By reading and experimenting, you'll eventually arrive at the right combination.

To see muscular definition in your abs, you should also follow a consistent program of aerobic exercise. By altering the body's chemistry, aerobic exercise helps the body break down fat for energy. Your ability to burn fat is optimized.

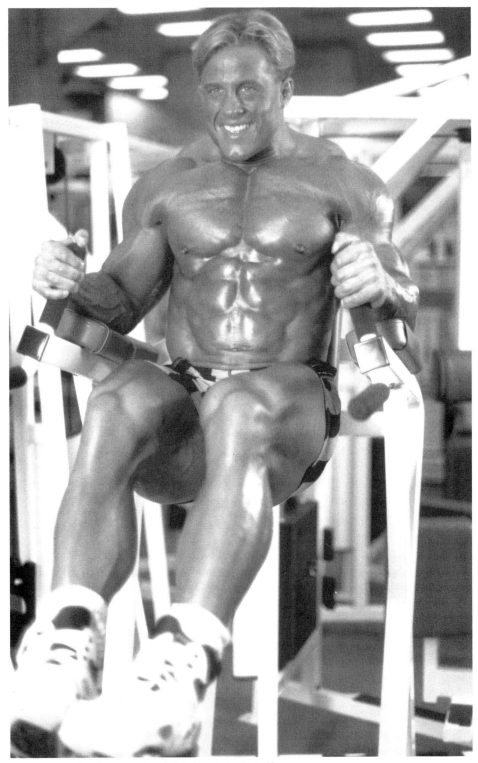

Knee-ups target the lower abs. *Photo by Irvin J. Gelb.*

30 SHAPING MUSCULAR ABS

Diet and aerobics trim the fat, while specific weight-training exercises tighten the muscles underneath. The primary muscle to target is the rectus abdominis (frontal abs). This muscle is worked by flexion—drawing the torso and the thighs closer together with exercises like crunches, leg lifts, and Roman chair sit-ups.

Avoid working the obliques, a muscle group that covers the sides of the midsection. Doing so only thickens the waist, unbalancing midsection proportions. Instead, concentrate on a muscle group called the serratus, located just above and to each side of your abdominals. Twisting leg raises target this area.

Nothing looks better than a tapered waist with ripped, hard abs. Here's a special routine that will give you those abs. Use it up to three times a week for best results. Stay strict on your nutrition program, too, so that your abs remain unobscured by body fat.

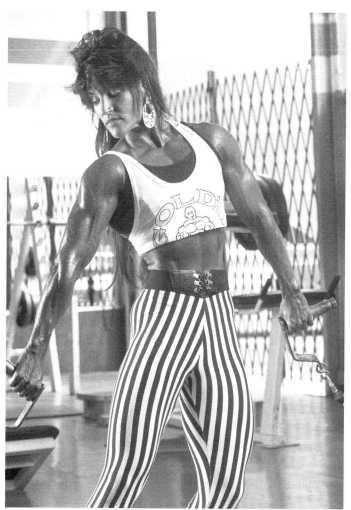

A tapered, tight waistline is the result of attention to diet, regular aerobics, and targeted ab training. *Photo by Ralph DeHaan.*

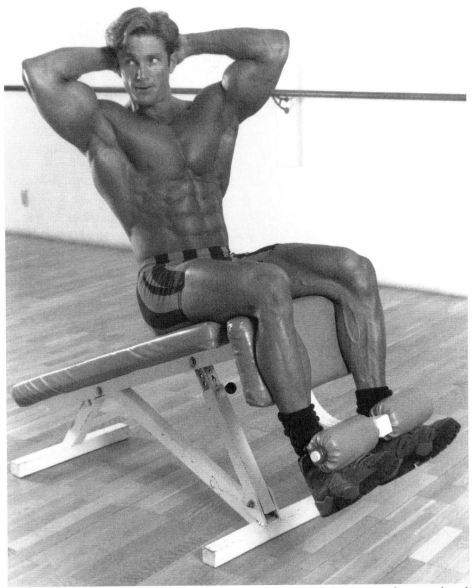

Using a slant board works abdominal muscles hard, as Lee Garoutte shows. *Photo by Irvin J. Gelb.*

Exercise #1: Abdominal Isolation Exercise. This is an exercise I developed specifically for isolating the abs. It requires a partner and a slant board.

Get into position by hooking your insteps under the padded roller or bar at the top of the board. Then have your workout partner lie facedown behind you on the slant board. Your partner's torso should abut your glutes. While forming a cushion for your lower back, this positioning secures your hip joint and isolates your abs.

Clasp your hands behind your head and lift your torso up toward your knees. Keep your ab muscles completely tight and retracted as you curl forward. Crunch down at the top. Using the strength of your abdominal muscles, pivot over your partner, not at your hip joint. Get a good stretch at the bottom of the movement. Do 2 to 4 sets of this exercise, with 20 to 25 reps each time.

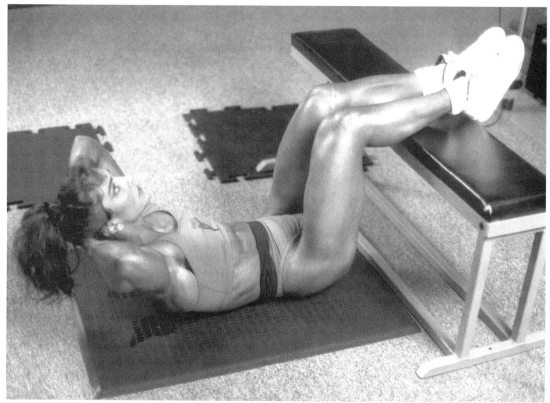

In any abdominal crunch exercise, it's important to keep your abs tight throughout the movement, as Laura Bass demonstrates. *Photo by Irvin J. Gelb.*

Exercise #2: Cable Crunch. This movement will really sharpen your lower abs, provided you do it properly. Take hold of the cable and tuck your hips forward to isolate your lower abs. Crunch down, while keeping your abdominal muscles tight. Lower your glutes to your heels to really isolate your lower abs. Do 2 to 4 sets, with 20 to 25 reps each time.

Exercise #3: Roman Chair Sit-ups. Sit in the Roman chair apparatus and lean back to a fully extended position so that your torso is below parallel to the floor. Get a good stretch in your abdominals as you lean back. Tightly crunch your abs to bring your torso up and forward. Do 2 to 4 sets, with 20 to 25 reps each time. If you have back problems, do not include this exercise in your ab training routine. Done incorrectly, it poses potential strain to the lower back.

Exercise #4: Twisting Leg Raise. Take hold of the bar. Bend your knees and hold them high in front of your body. Crunch up with your abs and twist your body slightly to one side and then to the other. Concentrate on proper flexion by contracting your abs, rather than just moving your legs. Do 2 to 4 sets, with 20 to 25 reps each time.

31 BUILDING A WIDE, RIPPED BACK

My views on training the lats have been well publicized, especially with regard to two key exercises—the pull-up and the lat pulldown. The standard pull-up is the most effective lat-building exercise that exists. No machine can ever take its place. Bodybuilders who try to build their lats on machines alone will be sorely disappointed with their lack of progress.

Make the pull-up the centerpiece of your lat training. When performing this exercise, bend your knees and hold them in front of your torso. This keeps your back from arching and isolates your lower lats, the segment of the muscle that displays most of the width. Another important point of technique is to pull your shoulders down at the top of the exercise and pull your elbows in close to your sides. This positioning subjects your lower lats to further stress.

Pull-ups are mass builders for the lats. But you need separation, too. To get the best of both worlds, superset pull-ups with pullovers. In other words, immediately after your set of pull-ups, do a set of pullovers, with no rest between the exercises.

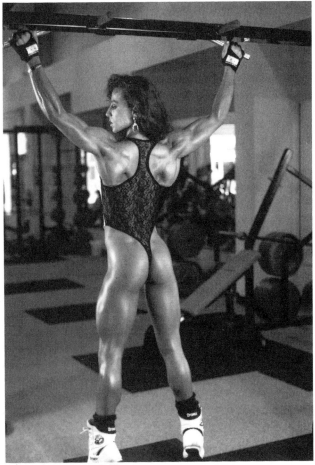

Wide-grip pull-ups. *Photo by Irvin J. Gelb.*

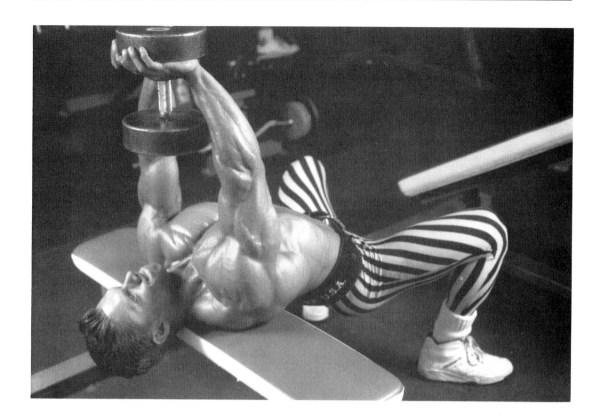

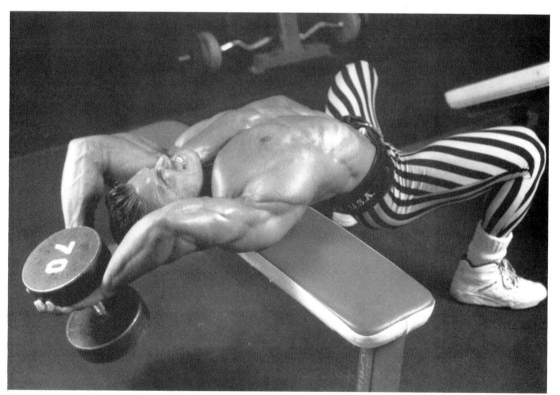

For mass and separation, superset pullovers with pull-ups. Vince Galante demonstrates proper technique from start to finish. *Photos by Irvin J. Gelb.*

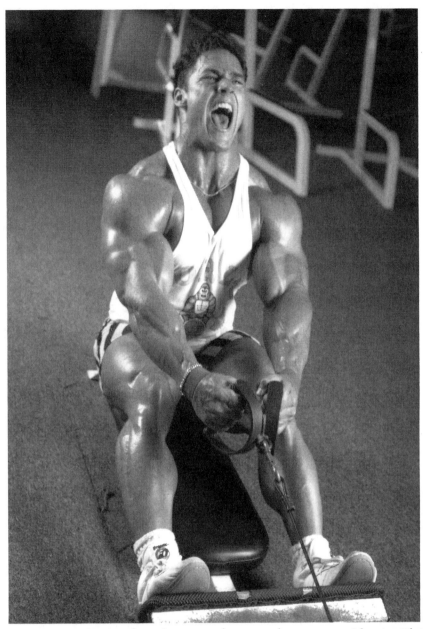

Use seated rows to perform exhaustion sets after your heavy pyramid sets. *Photo by Irvin J. Gelb.*

The pullover is a basic exercise best performed with a single dumbbell. Select a weight that is light enough to allow a deep stretch. With your body at a 90-degree angle to the bench, lie back with the weight behind your head. Press your shoulders down toward your waist and into the bench. Keeping your elbows slightly bent, pull the weight up over your head in an arc until it is positioned just above your chest. At this point, push your chest up and squeeze hard, pulling your shoulders down. Flex your abs and lock your elbows. Return to the starting position, arching your back slightly to stretch your rib cage. Perform 10 reps of pullovers in this manner. Follow these with a lat stretch at a piece of stationary equipment. (This fascial stretch is explained in section #14.)

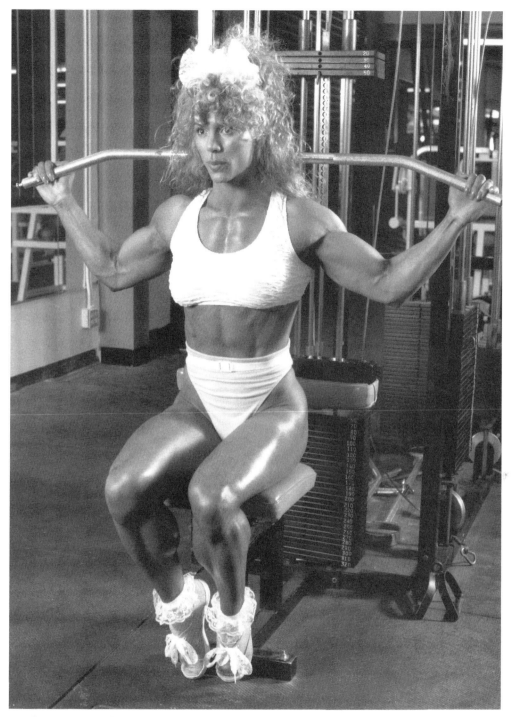

As Heather Tristany demonstrates, behind-the-neck lat pulldowns work the upper lats and the rhomboids. *Photo by Irvin J. Gelb.*

It's best to do 3 to 4 supersets of pull-ups and pullovers. From there, move on to wide-grip lat pulldowns performed behind the neck. With this exercise, pull your shoulders down as you start the exercise. As with pull-ups, keep your back straight. As you pull the bar down, move your elbows inward, pressing them against the sides of your body.

Every 2 out of 3 back workouts, start with the muscle that needs the most work, either your lats or your rhomboids (the muscles of the midback). For example:

WORKOUT 1 (LAT EMPHASIS)

Exercise	Sets & Reps
Pull-ups	Perform the first set without weight for 12 reps. On the next 3 sets, hang weight from your waist, using the pull-up harness. Increase the weight each time, striving for 8 to 12 reps on each of the 3 sets.
Pullovers (supersetted with pull-ups)	1 set of 10 reps.
Lat stretch	Hold for 10 seconds.
Wide-grip lat pulldowns	Perform 4 sets of 8 to 12 reps each, pyramiding your poundages each set.
Lat stretch	Hold for 10 seconds.
T-bar rows (This sequence hits the rhomboids.)	4 sets, 8 to 12 reps each time.
Bent-over rows	1 set of 12 reps. On the second set, increase the weight for 10 reps.

WORKOUT 2 (RHOMBOID EMPHASIS)

Exercise	Sets & Reps
Bent-over rows (Pyramid your poundages.)	Perform 4 sets of 8 to 12 reps each.
Lat stretch	Hold for 10 seconds.
Seated rows (Pyramid your poundages.)	Perform 4 sets of 8 to 12 reps each.
Lat stretch	Hold for 10 seconds.
Wide-grip lat pulldowns	Perform 4 sets of 8 to 12 reps each.
Lat stretch	Hold for 10 seconds.
Close-grip lat pulldowns	Perform 4 sets of 8 to 12 reps each.
Pullovers (supersetted with close-grip lat pulldowns)	1 set of 10 reps.
Lat stretch	Hold for 10 seconds.

32 TRAPEZIUS SPECIALIZATION

Visualize this flat, triangular muscle in terms of an upper trapezius and a lower. The upper portion originates along the spine at the base of the skull and inserts on the end of the clavicle (the collarbone). The lower portion extends from the spine to the scapula (down to the middle of the back).

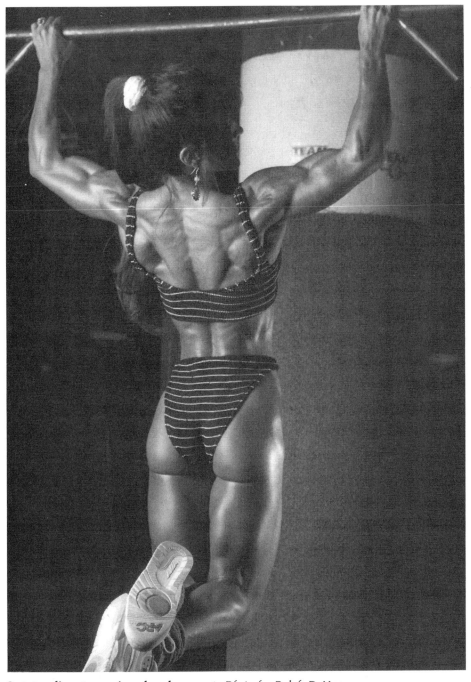

Outstanding trapezius development. *Photo by Ralph DeHaan.*

As multijoint movements involving the back, squats, deadlifts, and heavy behind-the-neck presses help develop the upper and lower trapezius. If you lag in development in this area, include shrugs in your routine. This exercise fully isolates the upper traps and can be performed with dumbbells, a barbell, or the bar of a bench press machine. Some pointers to get the most from shrugs:

- Lift the weights using the sheer strength of your traps, not by pulling with your arms.
- Some bodybuilders like to rotate their shoulder joint during the exercise. If you're in the habit of performing the exercise in this manner, you may want to reconsider your technique. Rotating the shoulder joint can take the stress off the traps.
- Squeeze your traps at the top of the movement.

Because the traps extend to the midback, make sure you're working this area as well—for a full center back. Now, you're probably thinking that there's got to be a "best" exercise to isolate the lower traps, just as shrugs are the best exercise for isolating the upper traps. But there's not. The best way to work the lower traps and the center back is by proper execution of behind-the-neck presses.

Most of the time, you see people performing this exercise at a seated bench as part of their delt routine. That's fine as long as they're not leaning against the back of the bench for support.

If you want even better results from this exercise—that is, bigger shoulders, thicker lower traps, and a full center back—do your presses without support, either in a standing position or seated at a flat bench. That way, you support the weight of your upper back by yourself, and your entire center back, including the lower traps, is called into play. To ensure proper back support, make sure you flex your abs at the top of the exercise. For additional performance tips on behind-the-neck presses, see section #35.

33 RHOMBOID DENSITY

The point of concentrating on rhomboid work is to build the center back. By far the most effective exercise for developing this area is the bent-over barbell row, as long as it's performed correctly. I've seen many bodybuilders with a shallow center back but well-developed shoulders, including rear delts. This gives the back an off-balance appearance and is usually a result of incorrect technique. There's a fine line between making the bent-over row a rear delt movement or a rhomboid exercise.

To begin, stand so that your feet are shoulder width apart. Take a wide grip on the bar to ensure that you work the rhomboids. A close grip creates greater arm and shoulder involvement. Bend over so that your back is parallel to the floor. Keep your back slightly arched.

Pull the bar up toward your chest while pushing your pecs down to meet the bar. In the contracted position, press your shoulders back and pinch your rhomboids together. If you omit this pinching action, you'll shift the leverage to your rear delts.

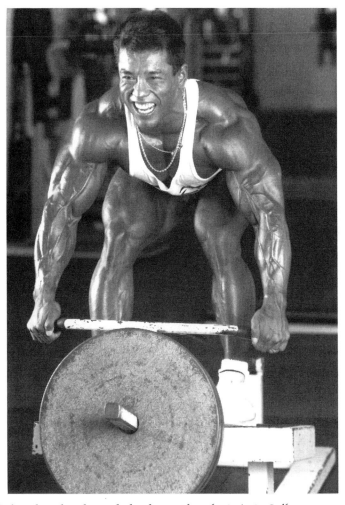

T-bar rows build the rhomboids and the lats. *Photo by Irvin J. Gelb.*

Here's an exercise sequence that will help you add thickness to your center back:

CENTER BACK ROUTINE	
Exercise	**Sets & Reps**
Standing behind-the-neck presses (Pyramid your poundages.)	Set #1: 12 reps Set #2: 10 reps Set #3: 8 reps Set #4: 6 reps
Bent-over barbell row (Pyramid your poundages.)	Set #1: 12 reps Set #2: 10 reps Set #3: 8 reps Set #4: 6 reps Exhaustion set: 15 to 20 reps
T-bar row*	Set #1: 12 reps Set #2: 10 reps Set #3: 10 reps Set #4: 10 reps Exhaustion set: 15 to 20 reps

* The T-bar row is an effective rhomboid-builder. It requires a special apparatus. To begin, take an overgrip on the handles and bend your knees slightly. Straighten your arms and arch your back. Keep your shoulders back during the movement. Pull the bar toward your chest. At the top of the exercise, squeeze your rhomboids and lower lats. Return to the initial position and repeat.

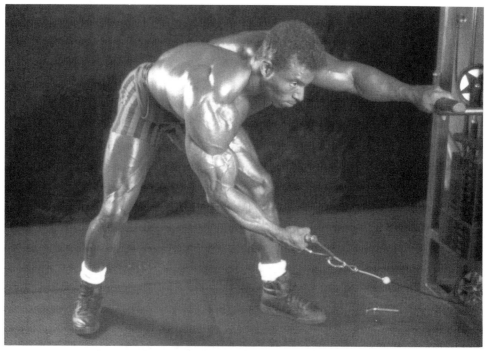

Cable pulley bent-over rows are an excellent exercise to use at the end of your back routine in a series of high-repetition exhaustion sets. *Photo by Irvin J. Gelb.*

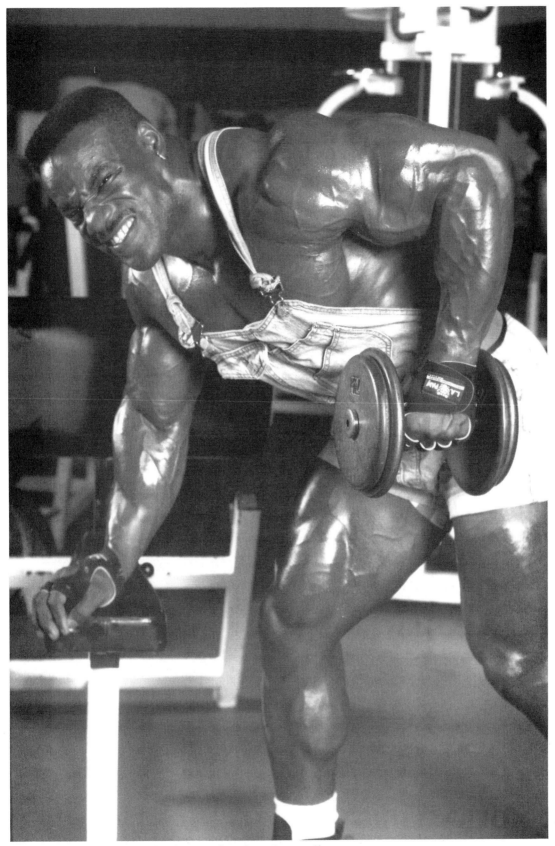

Chris Cormier goes for the burn. *Photo by Irvin J. Gelb.*

34 STRENGTHENING YOUR LOWER BACK

The muscles of concern in the lower back are the erectors. Think of them as two parallel columns that run along each side of the spine. Though most prominent in the lower back, the erectors span the length of the back and function as support structures for the spine.

A great deal of your ability to perform key building exercises such as squats depends on the strength of your erectors. If the erectors are weak or inflexible, low back pain or injury is often the result. As good insurance against this, you'd be wise to include some erector-strengthening exercises in your routine. Hyperextensions are one of the best.

Most people don't realize it, but a shift in body placement on the hyperextension bench can turn the exercise into a glute/hamstring isolation exercise. That's fine—if you want to firm up your glutes. But if stronger erectors are your goal, make sure you understand the correct positioning for this exercise. Here's what I mean:

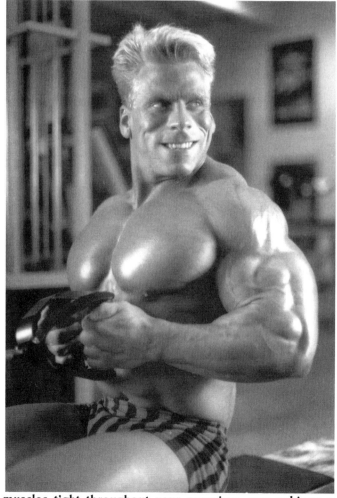

By keeping your muscles tight throughout your exercises, you achieve a more productive workout and make better gains. *Photo by Irvin J. Gelb.*

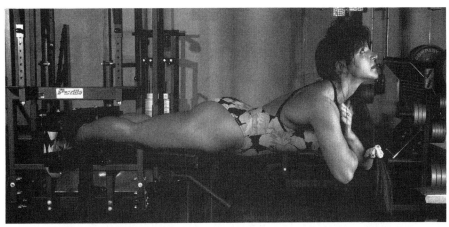

Performed correctly, hyperextensions strengthen the lower back. *Photo by Jimmie D. King.*

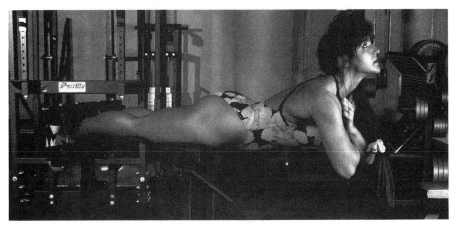

With hyperextensions, squeeze your erectors at the top of the exercise. *Photo by Jimmie D. King.*

A hyperextension bench has two components: a foot pad or roller that anchors your body and a small support pad for your lower torso. Hook your heels under the back of the foot roller and position your lower torso on the support pad so that you're free to pivot up and down at the hip joint. This position isolates the erectors. The farther forward on the support pad you position your lower torso, the more involvement your glutes will have.

As you begin the exercise, arch your back slightly and lift your torso upward. Squeeze your erectors at the top of the exercise. Lower toward the floor and repeat the exercise.

Another exercise to strengthen the lower back is the cable pull. It's a good exercise if you have injured your back. But check first with your physician, a qualified sports chiropractor, or a physical therapist before exercising an injured back.

All you need for this exercise is a piece of rubber cord such as surgical tubing. Sit on the floor and place the tubing behind your feet. Keep your knees slightly bent. Pivot forward, then come up with your back slightly arched. Press your abs out. Maintain constant tension on the muscles of the back.

As important as these special erector exercises is abdominal work, particularly crunches. Strong abs better support your spine and keep your back in proper alignment.

35 SHOULDER SHAPING

Few attributes of development are more impressive than an expansive shoulder line. That means large, well-shaped deltoids. The deltoid is a large triangular muscle that caps each shoulder. It gets its name from its resemblance to the Greek letter delta. The deltoid's main function is to lift the arm. It is assisted in this action by the pecs, the lats, and the teres major.

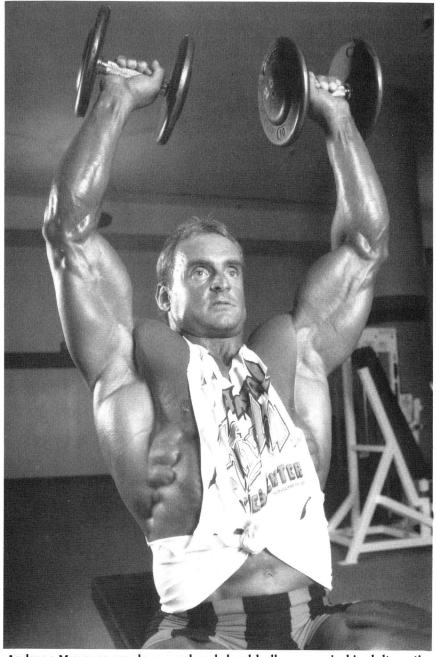

IFBB pro Andreas Muenzer employs overhead dumbbell presses in his delt routine. *Photo by Irvin J. Gelb.*

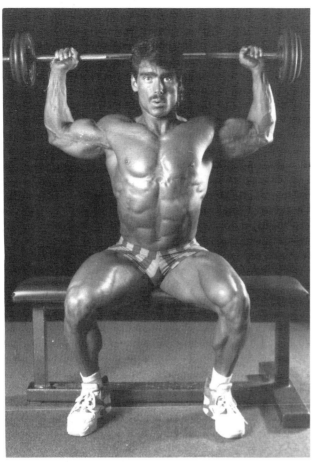

When performing behind-the-neck presses, avoid arching your back. Drop your shoulders and flex your lats as you press the weight upward. This action directly isolates your delts. *Photo by Irvin J. Gelb.*

Begin to think of the deltoid not as one muscle, but as three: the anterior (front delt), medial (middle delt), and posterior (rear delt). When designing a routine, select exercises that target each of these areas to maximize development of the entire deltoid. (For an example of how to design a routine for the delts, see section #42 on priority training.)

Both the front and middle delts are worked most effectively by pressing movements. The best exercise is the basic behind-the-neck press with a barbell. But the exercise isn't as important as how you perform it. A few key tips:

- While holding the bar in the overhead position, drop your shoulders and flex your lats. This puts the leverage on the delts, not the trapezius.
- Press the weight upward and lock your elbows. As you lock out, press your chest forward while tightening your abs. Then push the weight back slightly, but without arching your back or leaning backward. This action isolates your delts.

I prefer behind-the-neck presses to front shoulder presses for development of the entire front and middle delt area. With front shoulder presses, there's a tendency to arch backward during the exercise when the barbell is in the raised position. This takes the emphasis off the medial delts and limits the effectiveness of the exercise.

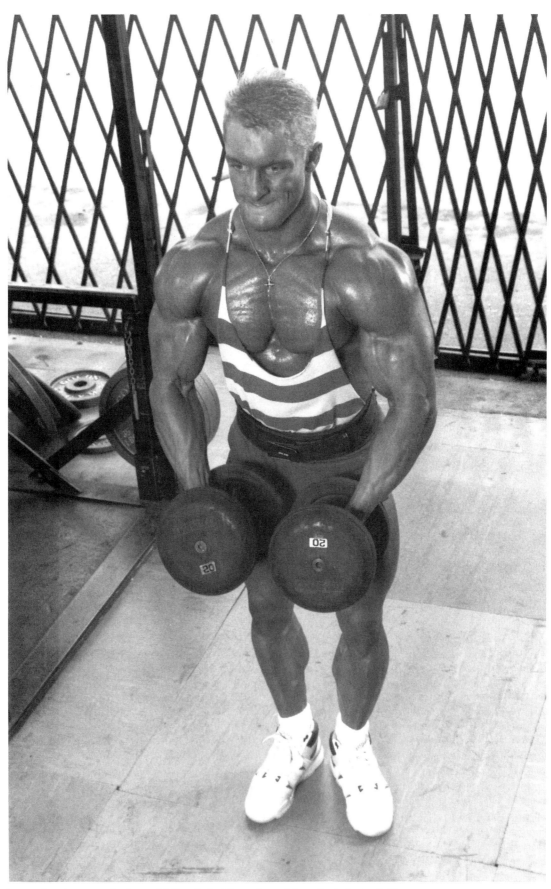

Lateral raises work the middle deltoid region. *Photo by Irvin J. Gelb.*

36 ADDING INCHES TO THE REAR DELTS

The standard behind-the-neck press works the rear delts, too. But if you want to really max out your rear delts, concentrate on another standard: rear lateral dumbbell raises. With a small adjustment in technique, you can make this exercise a great rear delt burner. I say this because many people do the exercise incorrectly. They bend forward and merely swing their arms upward, without really concentrating on the movement. This puts too much emphasis on the rhomboids and teres major and teres minor (two muscles located at the lower shoulder blade). Follow these steps, and you'll better challenge the rear delts:

- Grasp two dumbbells and bend forward so that your upper body is at about 30 degrees to the floor.
- As you raise the weights, bring your elbows slightly forward and up. This is the critical action for isolation. Then squeeze your delts.
- Raise the weights as high as you can for maximum rear delt involvement. Keep your elbows up. Notice a difference? Get a rhythm going as you execute each step in the performance of this exercise.

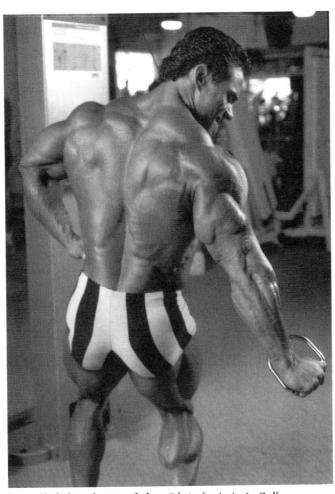

James Harrison has well-defined rear delts. *Photo by Irvin J. Gelb.*

37 BUILDING THE BICEPS PEAK

On many bodybuilders, you see either a prominent "biceps peak" or a large muscle "belly." The belly is the point about a third of the way down the arm where the two heads of the biceps converge. In well-developed biceps, there will be a split between the two heads before they come together. At this juncture, the outer head of the biceps may assume the shape of a small ball known as the "peak."

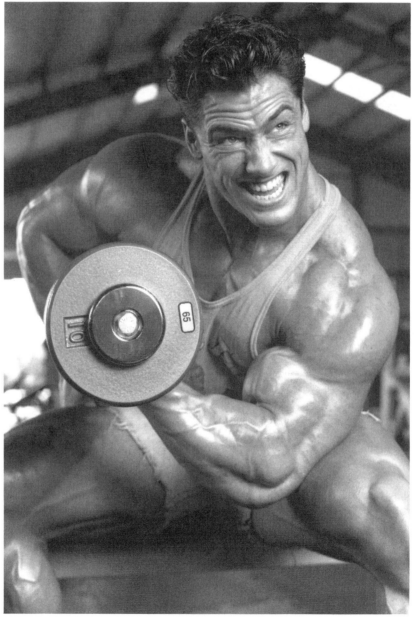

The concentration curl is another excellent exercise for building your biceps peak. *Photo by Irvin J. Gelb.*

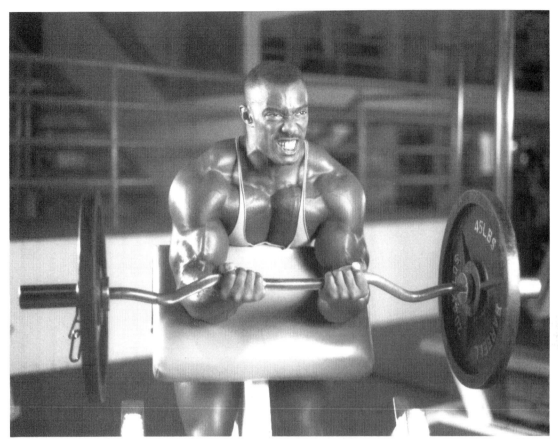

Beau Matlock begins a set of preacher curls. At the top of the exercise, pull your elbows together. This isolates your biceps and stimulates the muscles. *Photo by Irvin J. Gelb.*

A common lament among some bodybuilders is: "I can't build a biceps peak no matter what I do." Not true. You can—by using a few carefully chosen exercise techniques designed to work the outer head of the biceps.

One of the best exercises for developing a peak on your biceps is the biceps curl using an "EZ" or cambered curl bar. This bar lets you perform certain techniques that are important in the biomechanics of building a peak.

First, take a narrow grip on the bar. This places the emphasis on the outer head. Keep your shoulders down. If you lift them up as you curl, you bring your delts and traps into the exercise. That's counterproductive when you're concentrating on biceps.

As you lift the bar up, cock your elbows out slightly. Keep them in this position throughout the lifting and lowering phases of the exercise. By shortening your grip and angling your elbows out, you isolate the outer head of the biceps.

You can use some of the same techniques with dumbbell curls. As you begin this exercise, press your shoulders down. Curl up, using a "hammer curl" position in which the palms of your hands are turned upward (supinated) about 30 degrees. Toward the top of the curl, drop your shoulders and angle your elbows out slightly. You should feel the stress on your outer head.

PEAK-BUILDING ROUTINE

Exercise	Sets & Reps
EZ-bar curls (Pyramid your poundages.)	Warm-up set: 12 reps Set #1: 15 reps Set #2: 12 reps Set #3: 10 reps Set #4: 8 reps Exhaustion sets: 1 to 3 sets of 15 to 25 reps.
Biceps stretch	Hold for 10 seconds.
Dumbbell curl, using a hammer curl position (Pyramid your poundages.)	Set #1: 12 reps Set #2: 10 reps Set #3: 10 reps Set #4: 10 reps Exhaustion sets: 1 to 3 sets of 15 to 25 reps.
Biceps stretch	Hold for 10 seconds.

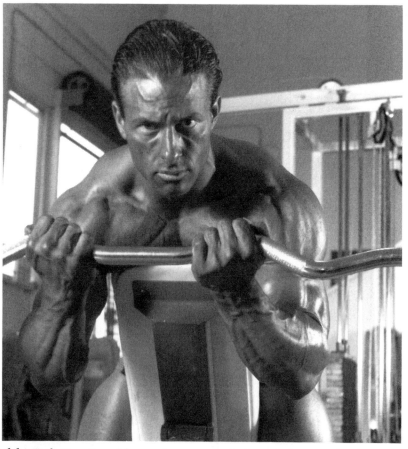

Demonstrated by Rob Russo, spider curls are a variation of the standard preacher curl exercise. To perform them, simply lean over the bench so that your arms point straight down. Your torso should be parallel to the floor. *Photo by Irvin J. Gelb.*

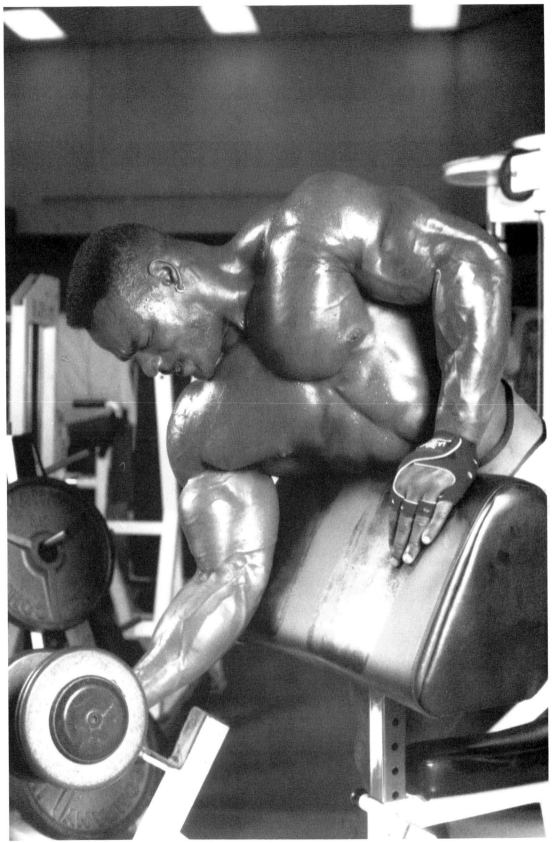

Spider curls can be performed with dumbbells, as Chris Cormier demonstrates. *Photo by Irvin J. Gelb.*

38 BOOST YOUR BICEPS MASS

For total development of your biceps, concentrate on movements that work the belly of the biceps in addition to those that stress the peak. As with exercises for the peak, grip length and arm positioning become critical.

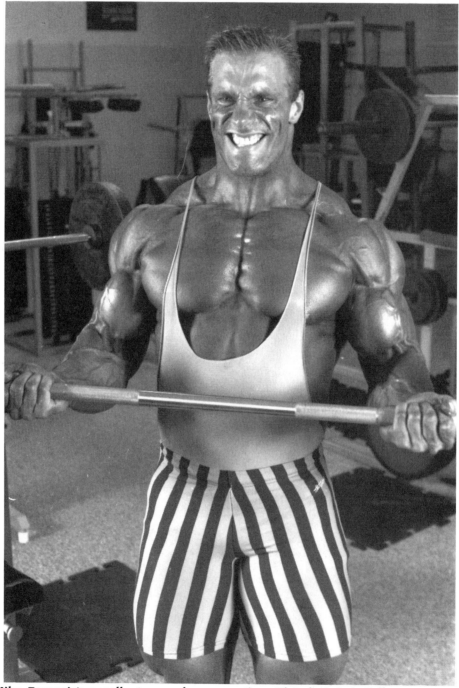

Note Mike Francois's excellent muscular separation. *Photo by Irvin J. Gelb.*

An excellent exercise for the belly is the barbell curl using a straight bar. To begin, take a wide grip on the bar—slightly wider than shoulder width.

As you lift the weight, literally drag the bar upward, keeping it close to your body. In the contracted position, pull your elbows in against your sides. Hold the weight for a count of 2. Then lower slowly, holding your biceps tight, and pull the bar back to the starting point with the strength of your triceps. This is a good habit to have on any type of curling exercise because it keeps constant tension on your biceps throughout the full range of motion.

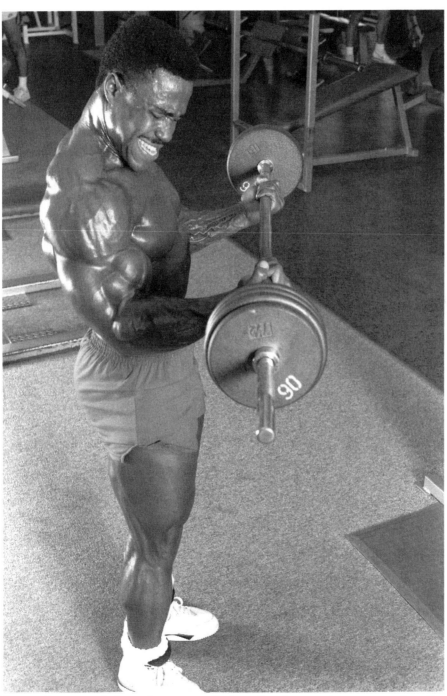

Mike Ashley performs curls in a slow, controlled motion for maximum muscular stimulation. *Photo by Irvin J. Gelb.*

The preacher curl is another exercise that works the belly effectively. You can perform preacher curls with a barbell, dumbbell, or cables. When curling the bar upward, move your elbows toward the center of the pad as if you were trying to make them touch each other. This action increases the tension on the belly of the biceps. Be sure to perform fascial stretching for the biceps between each exercise set.

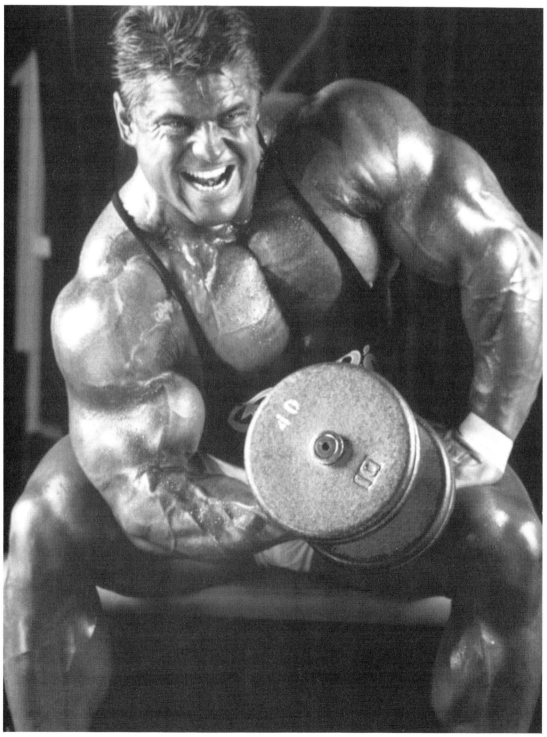

Keep every muscle tight when performing biceps exercises. *Photo courtesy of Eddie Robinson.*

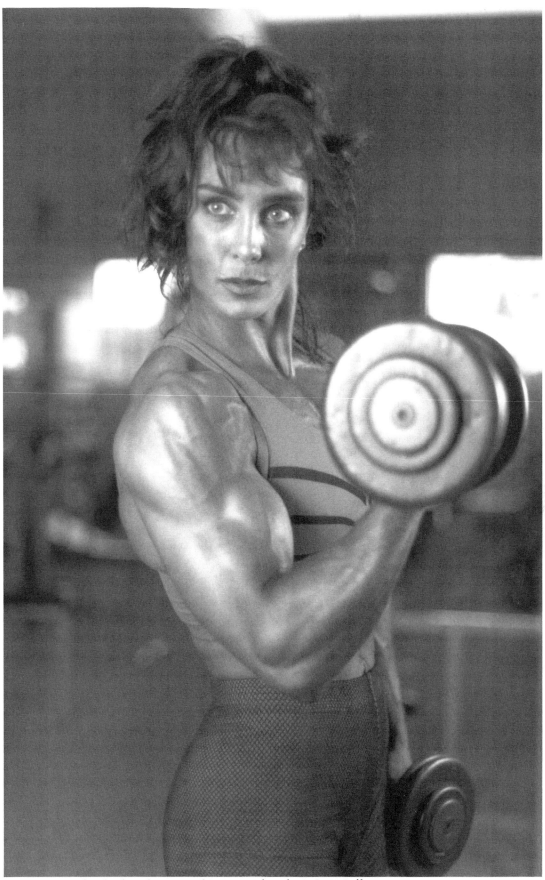

Laura Bass checks her form on this rep. *Photo by Irvin J. Gelb.*

39 REDEFINING YOUR TRICEPS

Three of the most effective exercises for working the three-headed triceps muscle at the back of the upper arm are barbell triceps extensions, triceps pressdowns, and close-grip bench presses.

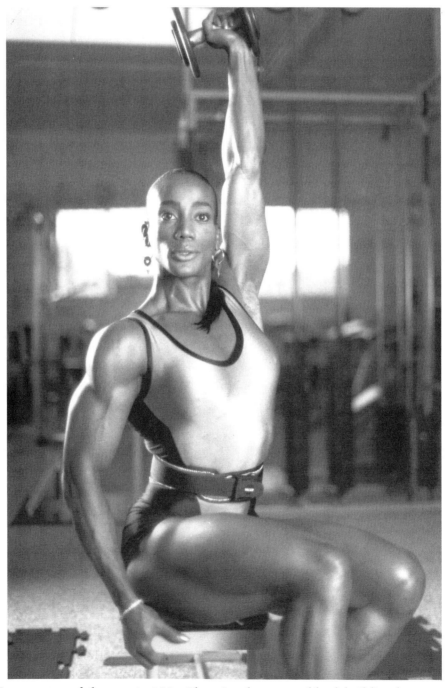

Lenda Murray—one of the greatest Ms. Olympias the sport of bodybuilding has ever known.
Photo by Irvin J. Gelb.

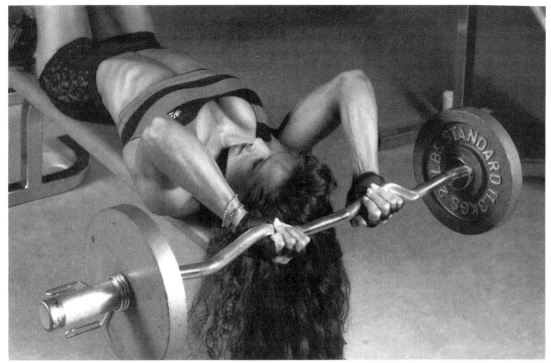

Moving the bar in an arc to the top of the bench is one way to perform lying triceps extensions. *Photo by Irvin J. Gelb.*

To correctly perform barbell triceps extensions, lie back on a flat exercise bench. Take a narrow (about six inches) overgrip on the bar. Extend your arms over your shoulders. Keeping your upper arms still throughout the exercise, flex your elbows and move the bar downward. At this point, you can work on shape or size, depending on how you guide the bar. For size, move the bar in a straight line, allowing your elbows to angle out. Keep your triceps tight and pull the bar down to a position just above your chin. Then push the bar back up to the initial position. The straight-line technique develops more of the belly of the triceps, resulting in greater mass.

For shape, move the bar in an arc, keeping your elbows pressed close to your upper body. This action works the "horseshoe" portion (the two outer heads of the muscle) of the triceps, leading to better shape of the overall muscle.

The same techniques can be applied to the triceps pressdown exercise, which uses a cable pulley attached to a weight stack. For mass, keep your upper arms and elbows close to the sides of your body as you press the bar down to a fully locked-out position. This technique, which I call the "strict method," targets the entire triceps muscle.

When you "cheat" the exercise—that is, angle your elbows out as you push through the exercise—you build the belly or third head of the triceps. Doing so adds better shape to the muscle.

With either version of the triceps pressdown, I recommend that you use a rope attachment or triceps handle attachment because they extend your range of motion. At the bottom of the exercise, you can press back farther, rather than stopping at a point limited by a bar. That way, you stimulate more of the muscle.

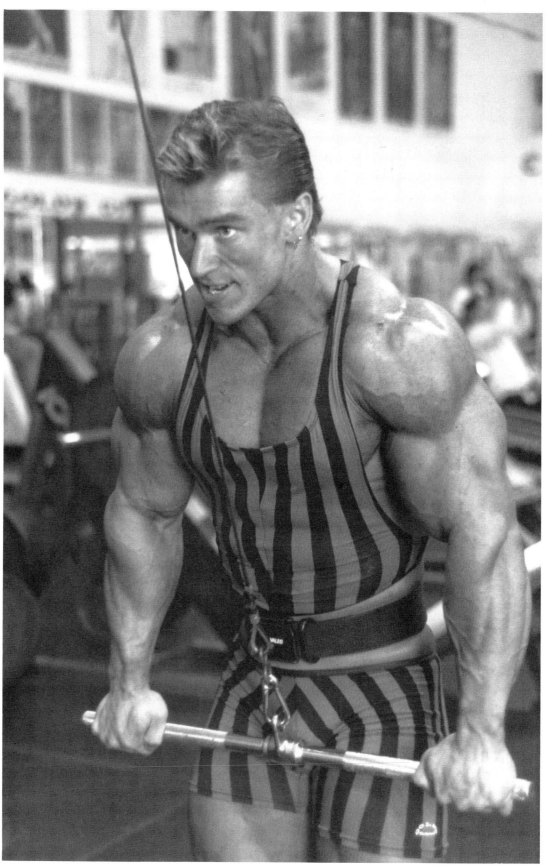

Note Lee Priest's excellent form as he keeps his upper arms and elbows pressed close to his body while strictly performing triceps pressdowns. *Photo by Irvin J. Gelb.*

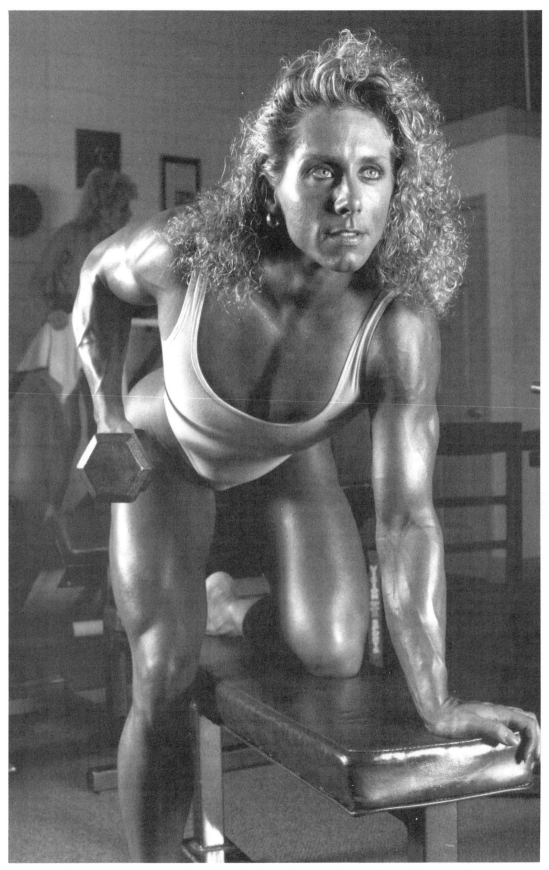

Jackie Rodgers begins a set of triceps kickbacks. *Photo by Irvin J. Gelb.*

Lock out on every rep to ensure that none of the muscle goes unworked. On the negative portion of the exercise, allow the strength of your biceps to pull the weight back to the starting point.

An exercise often employed to work the triceps is the close-grip bench press. To perform this exercise, lie back on a flat exercise bench and take a narrow overgrip (about six inches) on the barbell. Extend your arms so that the barbell is directly over your shoulders. From this position, bend your elbows and lower the bar so that it touches your upper pectorals. As you lower the weight, you must keep your elbows pushed up toward the ceiling to get the full effect of the exercise. This adjustment in technique isolates the triceps and takes stress off the pecs and the delts. In other words, the close-grip bench press becomes more of a triceps exercise, and less of a compound movement.

For best results in your triceps training, incorporate all of these techniques and exercise into your routine. The following routine can really be two routines in one, depending on how you perform your exercises. On your first triceps day of your training week, do the exercises using the "cheat method." On the next day of your triceps training, use the stricter method in which you keep your elbows in and pressed close to your body. Then alternate these routines from workout to workout.

TRICEPS ROUTINE

Exercise	Sets & Reps
Close-grip bench press (Pyramid your poundages.)	Warm-up set with an unloaded bar. 4 sets: 8 to 12 reps each set
Barbell triceps extensions—"cheat" style (Pyramid your poundages.)	4 sets: 8 to 12 reps each set
Triceps pressdown—"cheat" style	4 sets: 8 to 12 reps each set
Triceps kickbacks*	Exhaustion sets: 2 to 3 sets, 15 to 25 reps (Rep out to muscular failure.)

The next time you perform this routine, use the stricter method on barbell triceps extensions and triceps pressdowns. Be sure to stretch and pose between each set.

*The triceps kickback helps develop the upper part of the triceps at the shoulder tie-in. To perform this exercise, grasp a dumbbell in one hand and bend at the waist so that your upper body is parallel to the floor. Keep your upper arm pressed against your body. Drop your shoulders. From this position, extend your arm back and look out, keeping your elbow high throughout the exercise. Flex as hard as you can in the contracted position.

40 IMPRESSIVE FOREARMS— WITHOUT EXTRA EXERCISE

The forearm is a group of several muscles used primarily for arm extension and flexion. There are five major extensor muscles on the top portion of the lower arm. Together, these are responsible for extending the wrist. Located on the palm side of the forearm are three major flexor muscles used to bend the wrist forward. Strengthening all of these muscles, for greater power, is important in sports like tennis, racquetball, golf, and baseball. Strong forearms also help prevent injuries such as strains or sprains.

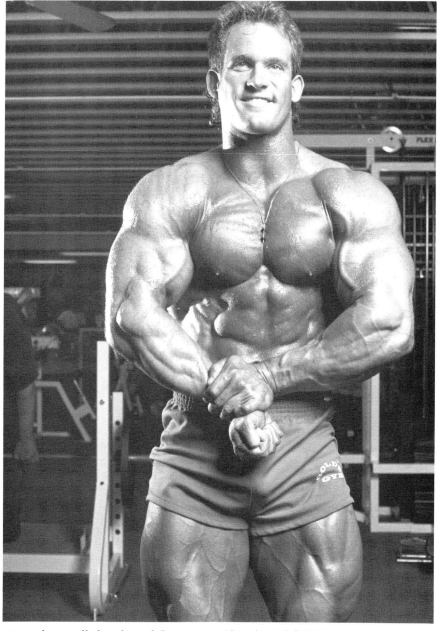

Note John DePolo's well-developed forearms. *Photo by Ralph DeHaan.*

If you're like most people, you probably don't think much about working your forearms. This is unfortunate because a well-developed forearm gives proportion to the total look of the arm. But before you start adding reverse curls or wrist curls to your routine, let me show you how to build forearms—without extra exercises.

First of all, kick the "strap habit." That's right. Don't wear wrist straps when you work out. Straps are typically used to supplement your grip so that it doesn't give out before you've finished a set. But straps are really a crutch. If you use straps all the time, you never strengthen your grip—or build your forearms. Show me a bodybuilder with weak forearms, and I'll show you someone who depends on straps.

The solution is to tighten your grip on exercises, particularly pull-ups, deadlifts, upright rows, and bent-over rows. As you lift the weight, tighten your forearm muscles and squeeze hard on the bar. A hard grip stabilizes the joint and, unlike a strap, builds the forearms.

Another important point is the positioning of your grip. Most people wind the palms of their hands all the way around the bar—a position that leads to friction and grip strain. A better grip is to cradle the bar in the first segments of your fingers. As you pull the bar to begin your exercise, tighten your grip, as explained above.

This method of gripping works very effectively with deadlifts. I never had big forearms until I started deadlifting as a competitive powerlifter. Once I progressed to lifting over 600 pounds—without straps—my forearms got huge. I'm not suggesting, however, that you have to deadlift 600 pounds to develop your forearms. Just forgo the straps and adopt a stronger, better-positioned grip on your exercises.

There's another secret to building better forearms—one you can try with the biceps curl. Hold the bar at the bottom of the exercise and curl your wrist back. Before lifting the bar up, curl your wrist forward. Then complete your normal curl. Incorporate this technique into your biceps curl routine. It makes the curl two exercises in one—one for the biceps and one for the forearms.

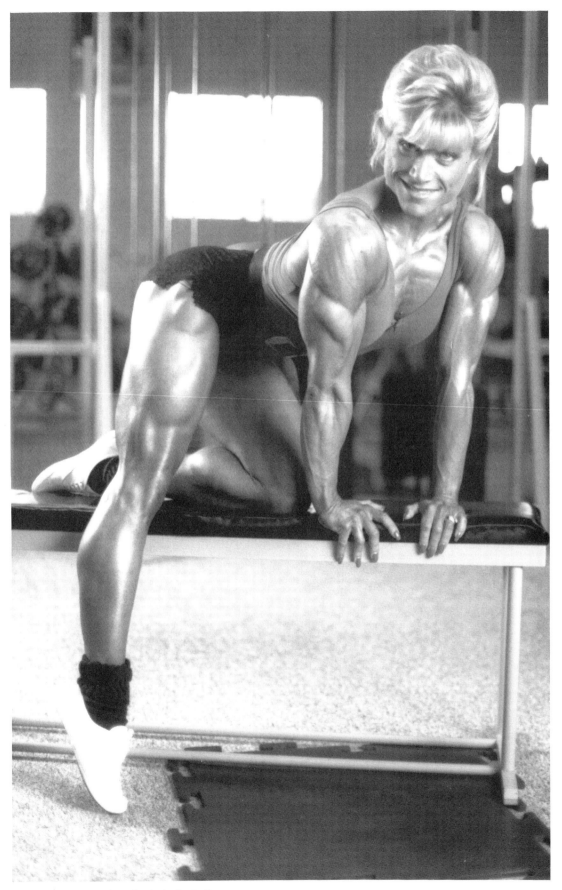

Drorit Kernes. *Photo by Irvin J. Gelb.*

41 ROTATION ROUTINES FOR ULTRA INTENSITY

Training routines come in many forms and variations. There's no single routine that works better than another. If your routine is producing results, then stick with it. Once you fail to get results, change your routine and examine your nutrition to make sure you're eating enough of the right kinds of foods.

The bodybuilders I work with train every day, often twice a day or more. Most people don't have that luxury, however. To approach the training frequencies of top-level bodybuilders, I suggest that you use a "rotation routine," dividing your body into sections and working certain body parts on separate days. A rotation routine is like a split routine—but with a difference. There's no rest day. If you need a rest day to recover so you can work out hard again, then you're spacing your body parts too close together, you're not eating enough quality calories, or you need to increase your nutrient density with supplements. When advanced, well-nourished bodybuilders take rest days, it's usually for personal obligations, not because they need to recover.

Here are three examples of rotation routines:

THREE-DAY ROTATION

Day 1	Legs and abs
Day 2	Chest and back
Day 3	Shoulders and arms
Day 4	Repeat the cycle.

FOUR-DAY ROTATION

Day 1	Quads and hamstrings
Day 2	Chest and triceps
Day 3	Back and biceps
Day 4	Shoulders, calves, and abs
Day 5	Repeat the cycle.

FIVE-DAY ROTATION

Day 1	Quads
Day 2	Back and hamstrings
Day 3	Biceps and triceps
Day 4	Chest and abs
Day 5	Shoulders and calves
Day 6	Repeat the cycle.

In selecting exercises for your routine, choose at least one basic exercise per body part: squats, belt squats, bench presses, pull-ups, behind-the-neck presses, and so forth. These should be the foundation of your workout.

When planning a routine, apply my suggested rep/set scheme, starting with low reps and heavy weight (pyramid sets) and finishing up with high reps and lighter poundages (exhaustion sets). Don't forget: Stretch and pose between every set.

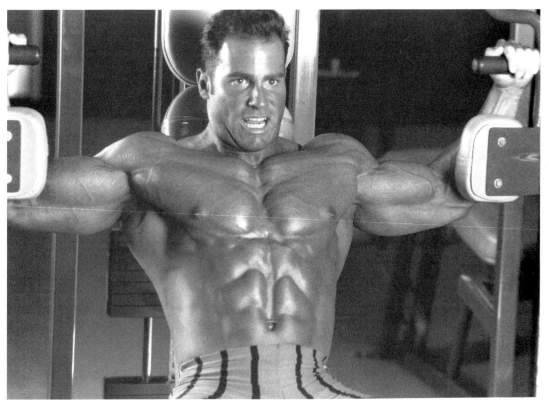

Flies performed on the pec deck machine work the entire pectoral, with emphasis on the inner pecs. *Photo by Irvin J. Gelb.*

42 PRIORITY TRAINING TO SHOCK STUBBORN MUSCLES

The techniques I've explained, along with combinations of exercises, can have a tremendous impact on muscular response. Add another factor to your workouts—priority training—and you'll tame lagging body parts once and for all.

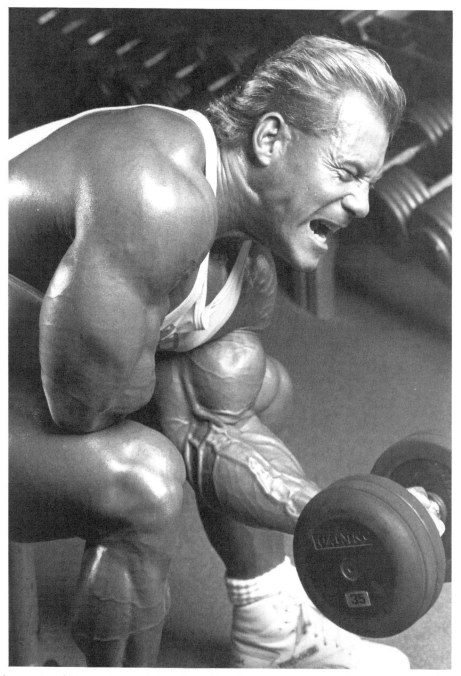

To build massive biceps, try training them first in your routine. *Photo by Ralph DeHaan.*

Priority training has to do with exercise order—training less-developed body parts first in a workout and training them harder, with more exercises, heavier weights, and higher repetitions.

Most explanations of muscle priority systems are based on an "energy rationale"; that is, train your most undeveloped muscles first in a workout, when you have the most energy. These routines are designed to allow body parts ample time to rest, so that no overtraining is involved and adequate time for recuperation is given.

This approach misses some fundamental points, however. If you're in a calorie surplus—that is, eating ample calories and taking in supplemental nutrients to support your energy needs throughout the day—then prioritizing based on energy and recuperation needs isn't required. Follow my high-calorie nutrition program, and you should have enough energy stamina to blast through any workout, regardless of how long or intense it is. You'll also have enough recuperative power to sustain you from workout to workout, without any compromise of energy.

Therefore, the first requirement of priority training is to put yourself in a calorie surplus so that you don't run out of energy, and you're well nourished enough to accelerate recuperation and promote muscular growth. In other words, if you want a muscle to grow, you have to eat enough to make it grow.

Fueled by being in a calorie-surplus state, you should next design a workout that puts lagging muscle groups at the top of the list. Let's say one of those lagging muscle groups is the deltoids, and you're working out on a three-day rotation. You'd schedule your routine like this:

Day 1: Deltoids, triceps, and biceps
Day 2: Legs, calves, and abs
Day 3: Back and chest
Day 4: Repeat the cycle.

You should increase your intensity on the delts by adding more exercises and increasing your workload on those exercises. Your delt routine might consist of four to five exercises instead of three. For example:

Exercise 1: Behind-the-Neck-Press. Use a barbell. Begin the routine with a warm-up set using an unloaded bar. Set your muscles up correctly by dropping your shoulders, then rotating them back as you press the bar up to an overhead position. Pyramid 4 heavy sets of behind-the-neck presses.

Exercise 2: Lateral Raises. Now it's time to blast each angle—your middle delt, front delt, and rear delt. Start with lateral raises for your middle delt. Grasp two dumbbells and position them at the sides of your body. Raise the dumbbells upward, keeping your elbows rotated back. At the top of the exercise (your arms should be raised to a point above shoulder level), lower your shoulders. This keeps the emphasis on the middle delt. Lower and repeat. Do 4 sets of these, pyramiding up on each set for about 10 to 12 reps each.

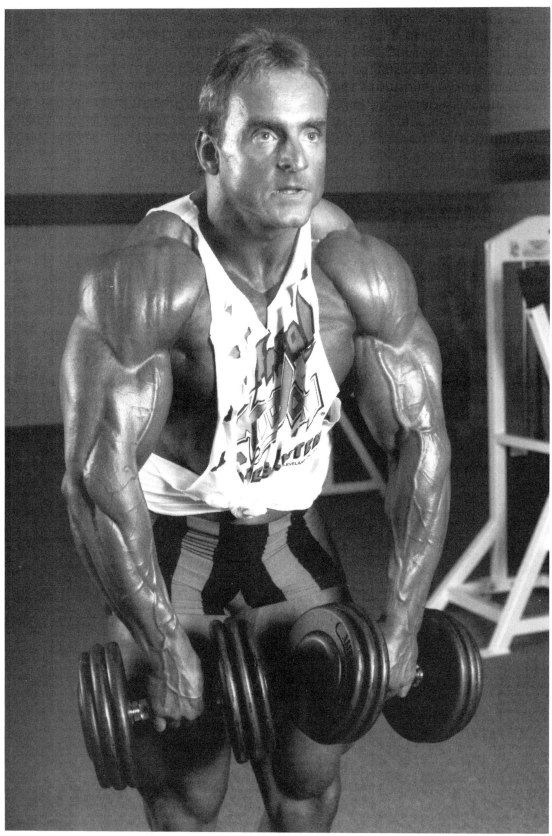

IFBB pro Andreas Muenzer. *Photo by Irvin J. Gelb.*

Exercise 3: Front Raises. In this exercise, you lift the dumbbells in front of your body, rather than to the side. Employ the same strict form as you did in the previous exercise. Again, do 4 pyramid sets.

Exercise 4: Rear Lateral Raises. Bend over at the waist until your upper body is about 30 degrees to the floor. Lift the dumbbells directly out to the sides until they reach shoulder level. Isolate your rear delt by keeping your shoulders pressed down. Don't pinch your shoulder blades in the contracted position; this will turn the movement into a back exercise. Perform 4 pyramid sets of rear lateral raises.

Exercise 5: Seated Strap Rows. Because of its "burn" effect, this cable exercise is an excellent exercise to perform as the exhaustion set portion of your routine. Using a wrist strap attachment, slip your hands through the loops of the straps. Twist both your elbows and the palms of your hands outward. With help from a partner, pull your elbows back as far as possible. Keep your shoulders down. As your arms come down, rotate them so that your arms face inward. Return to the starting position. Perform several exhaustion sets of 15 to 25 reps each.

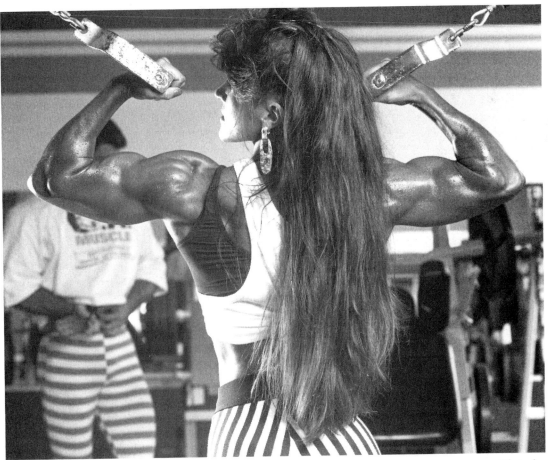

Cable curls are an excellent finishing exercise. Try them for your exhaustion sets. *Photo by Ralph DeHaan.*

A routine like this accomplishes three goals. First, you work each angle of the deltoids to ensure full development of the muscle. Second, the heavy poundages help accelerate growth. And third, the high-rep portion of the routine develops cardiovascular density. This refers to the expansion of your capillary network for more efficient delivery of nutrients to the muscles and better removal of waste products.

Any routine can be constructed in this manner to bring up weaker muscles. The key is proper nutrition, higher intensity, and greater workload—performed consistently from week to week until you achieve the desired results.

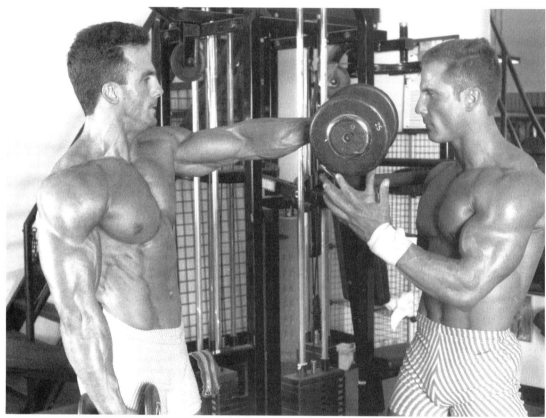

The use of a spotter is crucial to intense training. Shane McColgan (left) monitors Lance McColgan's form on front raises. *Photo by Irvin J. Gelb.*

43 STRENGTH TRAINING FOR MASS

If your problem is an overall lack of mass, rather than a lagging muscle group, a strength-training routine combined with a high-calorie, nutrient-dense diet may be the shortest route to greater size. Strength is the ability of a muscle to generate mechanical force and of the nerves to stimulate as many muscle fibers as possible. Strength training develops muscle fibers and trains the nerves running through them to discharge, or "fire," at once. With maximal stimulation of as many muscle groups as possible, you can build an excellent foundation of size and strength.

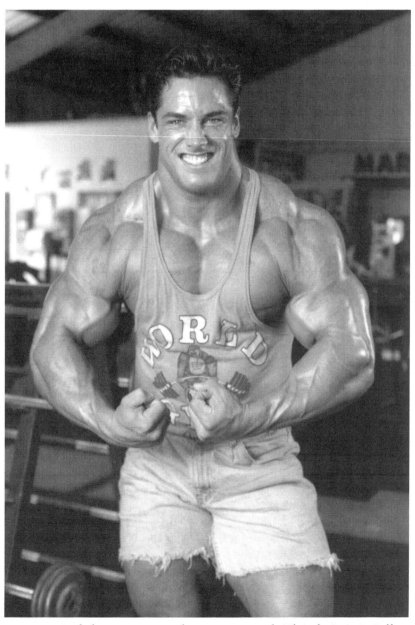

Dennis Newman—one of the most muscular guys around. *Photo by Irvin J. Gelb.*

There are several strategies to take. The first is the scientifically proven approach of following a heavy-poundage, low-repetition routine of basic exercises such as squats, deadlifts, bench presses, and overhead behind-the-neck presses. Three sets of 6 to 8 reps for each of these exercises have been shown to produce significant gains in a relatively short time (within about six weeks).

At a more advanced level, you can incorporate negative training into your workout to build greater strength. Negatives build a muscle in which more fibers fire at once. This activates muscular growth by stimulating a greater number of muscle fibers during muscular contraction. With negative training, you perform only the lowering portion of the exercise. Take the bench press, for example. Have your partner raise the bar up for you. Then lower it, while resisting the gravitational pull. In the training sequence, employ negative repetitions after you have completed your heavy pyramid sets.

Another advanced strategy is the use of forced reps in your routine. A forced rep is the continuation of a repetition after you've reached failure on an exercise. It requires the assistance of a training partner who gently lifts the weight just past your sticking point. From there, you take over, pushing the rep to completion. Using the bench press as an example again, here is a system for incorporating forced reps into your routine:

Advanced Bench Press Routine with Forced Reps

Set #1	10 to 12 reps
Set #2	8 to 10 reps
Set #3	6 to 8 reps
Set #4	4 to 6 reps, followed by 2 to 4 forced reps
Set #5	2 to 4 reps, followed by 2 to 4 forced reps
Set #6	1 rep maximum, followed by 1 to 2 forced reps
Set #7	Several forced reps

Notice that the above routine incorporates a 1-rep maximum, also known as a "single." Any low-rep scheme employing singles, doubles (2-rep maximums), and triples (3-rep maximums) has a definite strength-building effect. One reason is that low reps strengthen your connective tissue and help increase your Golgi tendon reflex (GTR) threshold. As explained earlier, this is a strength factor that determines your ability to sustain strenuous, high-intensity workouts. It is desirable to have a high GTR threshold. This means you can handle heavier weights and complete more repetitions without your Golgi tendon organs firing too soon. The higher your GTR threshold, the heavier and more intensely you can train. Intensity leads to greater gains in strength and size.

With each of these strategies, it's imperative that you stretch between sets (fascial stretching). Stretching in this manner also increases your Golgi tendon reflex threshold, resulting in strength gains of 15 to 20 percent.

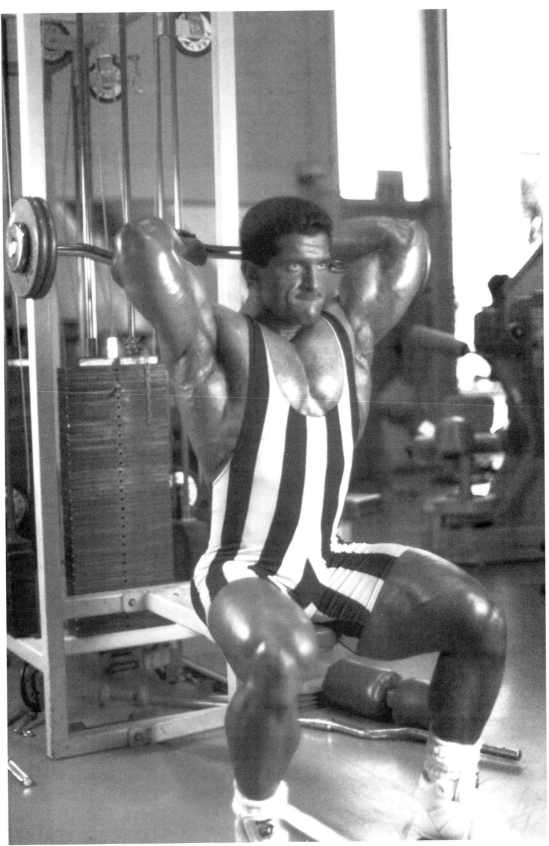

Bodybuilder Joe Spinello. *Photo by Irvin J. Gelb.*

44 POWERLIFTING CYCLES FOR BODYBUILDERS

Power training—low-rep/heavy-weight work with basic, compound exercises—is one of the quickest routes to building strength and mass. A drawback of this type of training, however, is that it leaves out high-rep work, which is so critical for building cardiovascular density and stimulating growth hormone release.

There are two effective ways to combine high-rep work with pure power training. Using basic power exercises, one way is to train in the 4-to-8-rep range one week and in the 12-to-20-rep range the next. For example:

First Week*

Monday/Exercises	Sets & Reps
Squats	Begin with a warm-up set. Pyramid the next 4 sets, using heavy poundages, for 6 to 8 reps each set.
Bench press	Begin with a warm-up set. Pyramid the next 4 sets, using heavy poundages, for 6 to 8 reps each set.
Triceps pressdown	Perform 3 pyramid sets, for 6 to 8 reps each set.
Straight-leg deadlift	Begin with a warm-up set. Pyramid the next 4 sets, using heavy poundages, for 6 to 8 reps each set.

Tuesday/Exercises	Sets & Reps
Behind-the-neck press	Begin with a warm-up set. Pyramid the next 4 sets, using heavy poundages, for 6 to 8 reps each set.
Biceps curl with a barbell	Perform 3 pyramid sets, for 6 to 8 reps each set.
Lat pulldown	Begin with a warm-up set. Pyramid the next 4 sets, using heavy poundages, for 6 to 8 reps each set.
Pull-ups	3 to 4 sets, 8 reps each

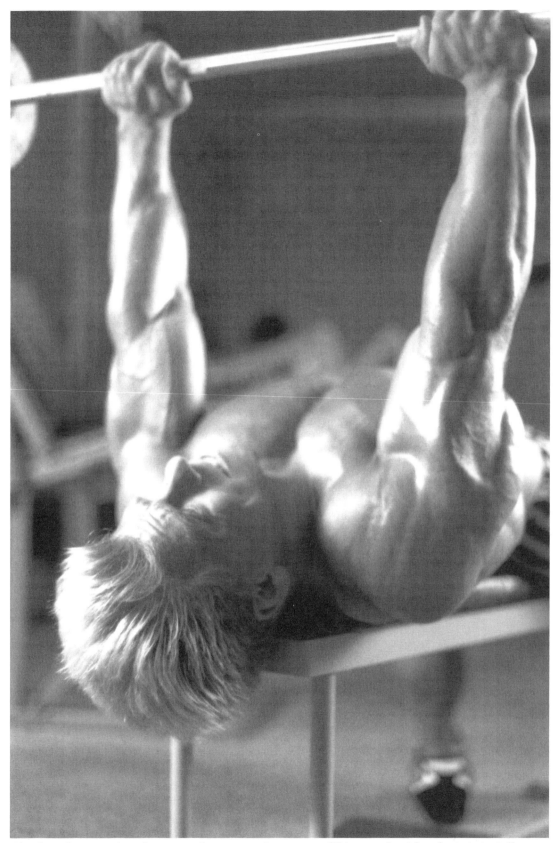

The bench press is a key exercise to use in a powerlifting cycle. *Photo by Irvin J. Gelb.*

Thursday/Exercises	Sets & Reps
Bench press	Begin with a warm-up set. Pyramid the next 4 sets, using heavy poundages, for 6 to 8 reps each set.
Close-grip bench press	Perform 3 pyramid sets, for 6 to 8 reps each set.
Regular deadlift	Begin with a warm-up set. Pyramid the next 4 sets, using heavy poundages, for 6 to 8 reps each set.
Squats	Begin with a warm-up set. Pyramid the next 4 sets, using heavy poundages, for 6 to 8 reps each set.
Shrugs	Perform 3 pyramid sets, for 6 to 8 reps each set.

Friday/Exercises	Sets & Reps
Behind-the-neck presses	Begin with a warm-up set. Pyramid the next 4 sets, using heavy poundages, for 6 to 8 reps each set.
Seated rows	Begin with a warm-up set. Pyramid the next 4 sets, using heavy poundages, for 6 to 8 reps each set.
Pull-ups	3 to 4 sets, 8 reps each
Dumbbell curls	Begin with a warm-up set. Pyramid the next 4 sets, using heavy poundages, for 6 to 8 reps each set.

* The next week, follow the same routine but increase the number of reps to 12 to 20.

Another strategy is to follow a "powerlifting cycle" involving heavy, low-rep work for four to six weeks. This period is followed by a "bodybuilding cycle," in which you train with moderate weights and higher reps for the next four to six weeks.

Both training methods combine the best of the bodybuilding and powerlifting worlds. Not only that, they help you break out of training slumps.

It's important to train intuitively, listening to your body and letting it be your guide to what levels of intensity you can handle during a particular workout. If a poundage feels heavy, for example, lower it and strive for more repetitions. Or if a weight feels too light, increase your poundages and go as heavy as you can. The key is to find what your body needs and can accomplish during each training session.

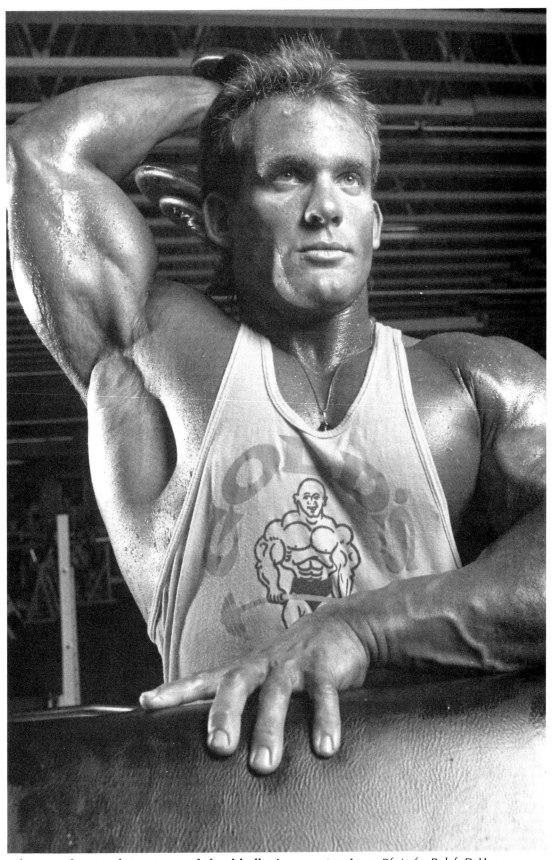

John DePolo completes a rep of dumbbell triceps extensions. *Photo by Ralph DeHaan.*

45 TENDON TRAINING

Tendons are thick, fibrous tissue connecting muscles to bones. The strength of your muscles is limited somewhat by the strength of your tendons—the amount of force they can handle during weight training. If the tendons are weak, your muscles will shake and eventually give out during a set. This is related to your Golgi tendon reflex (GTR) threshold, a protective response to overstretching a weight-bearing muscle.

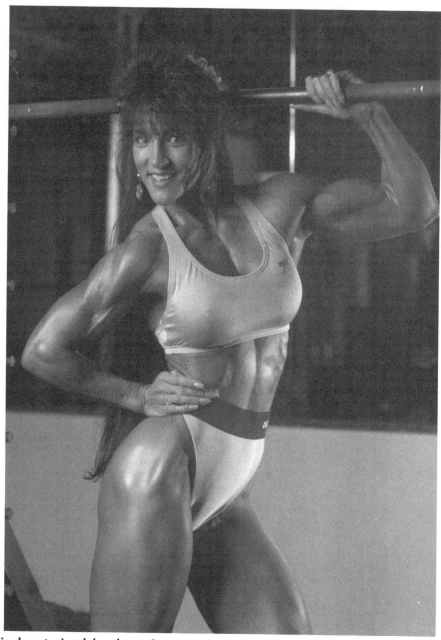

Lisa Lorio has trained hard—and smart—for this well-chiseled symmetry. *Photo by Ralph DeHaan.*

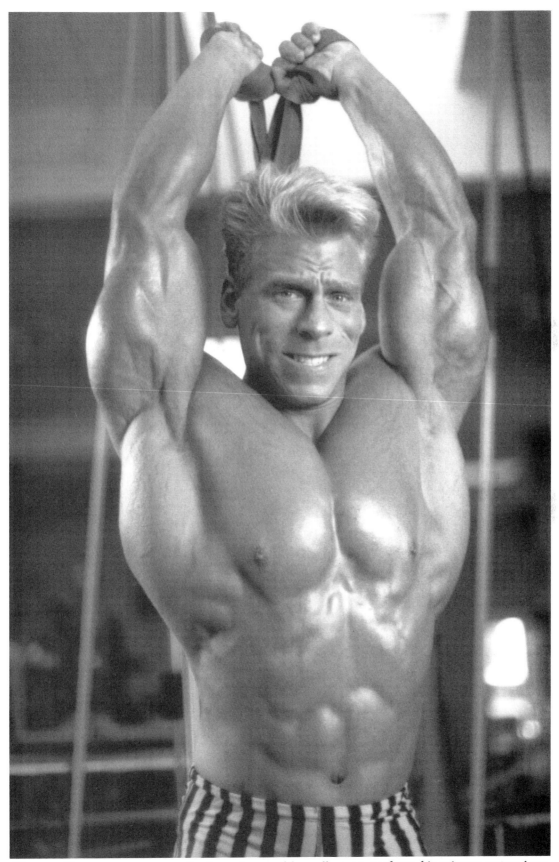

Thomas Varga uses a rope attachment on cable pulleys to perform his triceps extensions.
Photo by Irvin J. Gelb.

By strengthening your tendons and increasing your GTR threshold, you can lift heavier poundages. That translates into greater strength and size. Another advantage of stronger tendons is injury protection. Tendons are more prone to injury than muscles. Anatomically, tendons have a smaller cross section than muscles do, so force isn't distributed well. Moreover, tendons are situated in easily injured, unprotected areas of the body, where they rub against tissues like bones, ligaments, and other tendons. Some of the most common sports injuries involve "tendinitis," an inflammation of the tendon. Depending on the sport, common sites of injury are the Achilles' heel, the shoulder, and the elbow.

Certain training techniques will strengthen your tendons. One method is to incorporate "speed training" into some of your large-muscle (compound) exercises. The deadlift is a good example. On the last 2 reps of each set, when you're partially fatigued, perform the movement explosively—as quickly as possible—while still maintaining control over the weight. This will help condition your tendons. Another conditioning technique is to use heavy negative and heavy forced reps in your training.

TENDON TRAINING ROUTINE

Exercise	Sets & Reps
Deadlift (Perform the last 2 to 3 reps of each set explosively.)	Warm-up set: 20 reps Set #1: 15 reps Set #2: 12 reps Set #3: 10 reps
Bench press (Perform the last 2 to 3 reps of each set explosively.)	Warm-up set: 12 reps Set #1: 10 reps Set #2: 8 reps Set #3: 6 reps Set #4: Rep out to failure. Then have your partner assist you with several forced reps or negatives.

A consistent program of stretching between exercise sets (fascial stretching) will also improve tendon strength and conditioning.

46 MAXIMUM MUSCLE STIMULATION

Many people merely go through the motions on their last set. Your last exhaustion set is the time to give it all you've got—and stimulate the muscle even more. During this set, lower the weight slowly, emphasizing the negative portion of the exercise. This becomes especially important at the end of a set when the ATP in the muscle (the fuel that makes muscles contract and relax) is depleted. When a muscle runs out of ATP, it "locks up" in the contracted state and can't relax properly. This condition is known as "ischemic rigor."

When the muscle is in rigor as you are lowering the weight from the contracted position, the fibers can't relax, and they literally get torn as the muscle elongates. If this sounds painful, it is. Most people stop a set just as this occurs, because the pain is unbearable. But those who fight against the pain and crank out a few more reps are the ones who develop bigger muscles. Sorry, but that's the way it is!

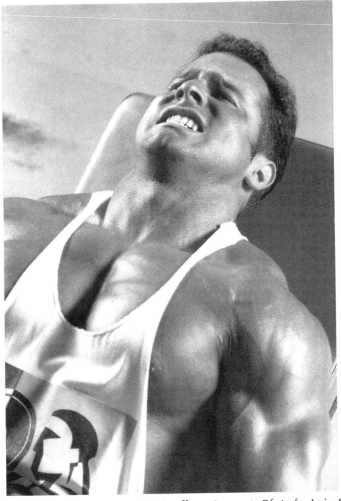

Your last exhaustion set is the time to give it all you've got. *Photo by Irvin J. Gelb.*

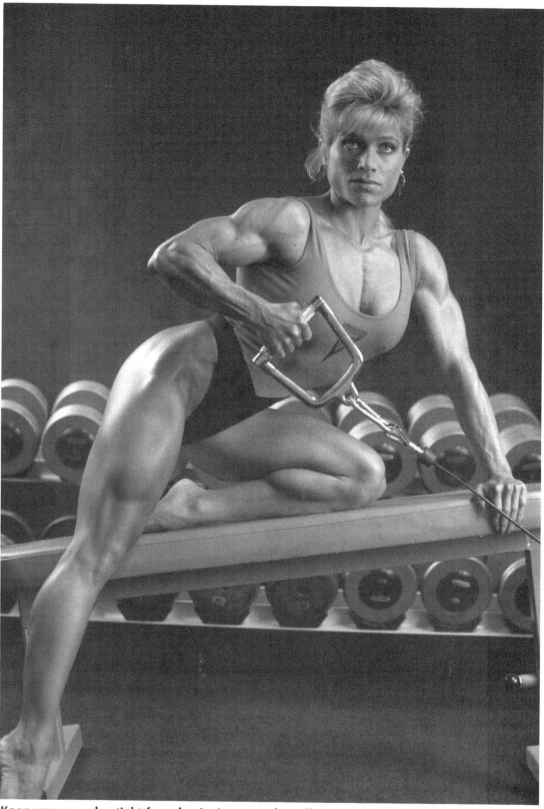

Keep your muscles tight from beginning to end in all your exercises. *Photo by Ralph DeHaan.*

47 INJURY-FREE TRAINING

A major contributor to sports injuries today is inadequate nutrition. Athletes, bodybuilders included, aren't matching their nutrition to their level of training. While training hard, they fail to recover properly from their workouts. The reason? They haven't increased their calories from nutrient-dense foods and supplements. Undernourished, their bodies simply can't handle the overload of hard training, so they wind up with injuries. In short, you're less likely to suffer from injuries if your nutrition and supplements match your training loads.

Another factor in injury prevention is flexibility—being able to move your joints over an allowable range of motion. Without flexibility, you're at risk for any number of injuries, including:

- Muscle pull. This is an acute tear in muscle fibers, characterized by a sudden sharp and persistent pain in a specific area of the muscle. Continuing to exercise will further damage the muscle fibers and aggravate the injury.

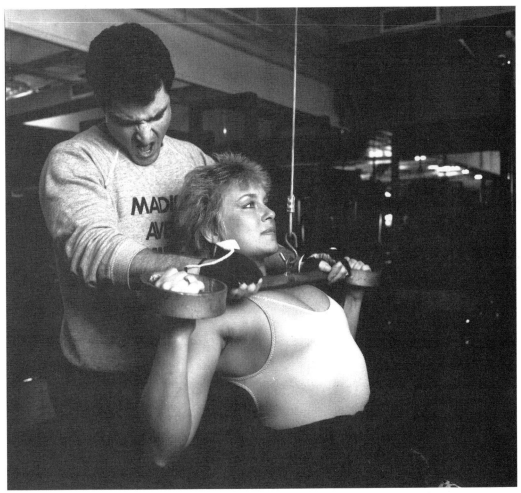

Trainer Patrick Arnao and bodybuilder Doris Powell. *Photo by Paul B. Goode.*

- Tendon rupture. Tendons attach muscles to bones. Ruptures in these fibrous bands of tissue can occur as a result of sudden contractions. There is a pop, and severe pain sets in. The affected area may become swollen, possibly with internal bleeding seen under the skin.
- Sprain. This is a rip in the ligaments, the connective tissue that holds your bones together. Ligaments are fairly elastic, but if stretched too far—more than 6 percent of their length—they snap, and you have a sprain. Severe sprains in which the ligament is torn completely apart often require surgery.

Good flexibility reduces your potential for injuries. The best way to increase flexibility is through fascial stretching. This conditioning technique gives your muscles and the joints they connect greater range of motion. A supple, flexible body can better withstand physical stresses. Stretching also helps prevent muscle soreness and promotes better recovery.

With any kind of surgery, it's critical to see a sports medicine physician, a qualified sports chiropractor, or a physical therapist, especially if the pain persists. Unless you seek prompt medical treatment, you could retraumatize the injury, causing it to become chronic.

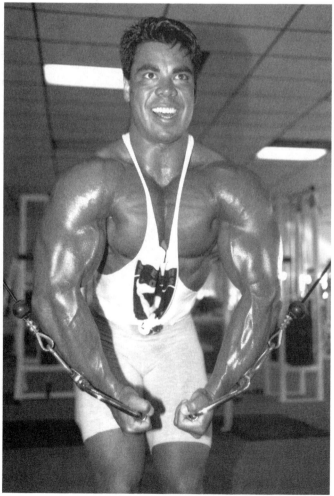

Proper technique helps prevent injuries. *Photo by Irvin J. Gelb.*

48 BREAKING PLATEAUS

If you've reached a plateau—a point at which you are not gaining any muscle—then you may not be taking in enough nutrients to support further growth. While maintaining a strict diet of lean proteins and complex carbohydrates, up your calories at the rate of 300 to 500 a day, so you gain up to one pound a week. Use medium-chain fatty triglycerides (MCT oil or MCFA oil) and protein/carbohydrate supplements to increase your calories. By doing so, you speed up your metabolism so that your body starts building muscles and burning fat more efficiently.

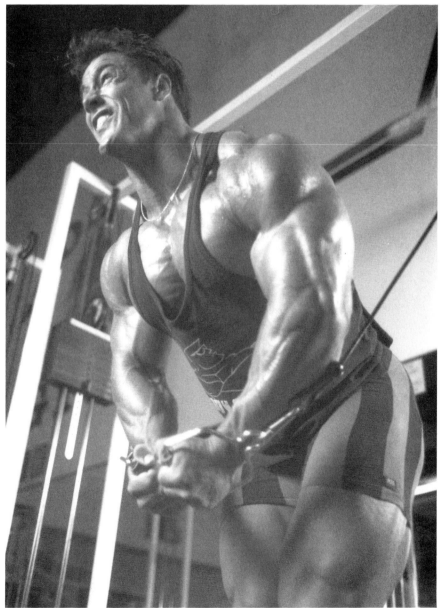

For size and shape, fight the pain and crank out a few more reps. *Photo by Irvin J. Gelb.*

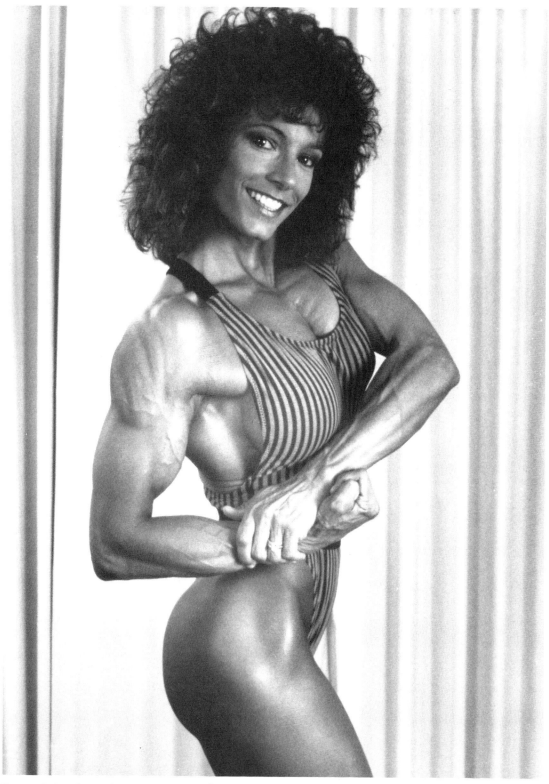

Penny Price is an inspiration to millions of women. *Photo by Jimmie D. King.*

Many bodybuilders who reach a plateau try to pack on muscle by following killer workouts. That's fine, as long as you're taking in enough quality nutrients and calories. But if proper nutrition isn't there to help you recover, those workouts won't do any good. Once you get in the habit of making your nutrition as intense as your training, you'll start growing in no time.

Not long ago, I worked with a state- and national-level title holder whose previous record body weight was 217, with 10 percent body fat. By gradually increasing his calories to 9,500 a day over a four-month period and incorporating aerobics and fascial stretching into his training program, he upped his weight to 233, with only 8.2 percent body fat—quite an improvement. Before then, he had never put on more than 4 pounds of muscle a year.

As this competitor learned, another way to break a plateau is with aerobic exercise. Many bodybuilders, however, typically shy away from aerobics, particularly in the off-season, fearing that it will cause a loss of muscle mass. This loss, however, has less to do with aerobics and more to do with improper diet. A bodybuilder who loses muscle during a period of aerobic training is simply not eating enough to compensate for the calories spent by the aerobic activity. Take in enough quality calories, and you'll preserve muscle mass while your body fat drops.

Aerobics forces oxygen through your body, increasing the number and size of your blood vessels. Blood vessels are the supply routes that transport oxygen and nutrients to muscles and other body tissues and carry waste products away. As mentioned earlier, the expansion of this circulatory network is called "cardiovascular density," and it's critical for muscular growth, repair, and recovery.

Here's why: Your ability to build additional muscle is limited by your degree of cardiovascular density. Without aerobics in your total bodybuilding program, your body can't create any additional supply routes necessary to feed the muscles. But the more blood vessels you have and the bigger they are, the more nutrients your tissues can receive to support growth and repair. That translates into longer, more intense workouts and, ultimately, bigger muscles.

Do your aerobics every morning for 45 to 60 minutes—before breakfast. At that time, your glycogen stores are low, because you've gone all night without eating. With glycogen in short supply, you begin burning fatty acids for energy. You become leaner as a result. Later, the nutrients you eat, including natural, starchy carbohydrates, are efficiently resupplied to muscles, without being turned into body fat, and your metabolism is activated for the entire day.

There are many types of aerobic activities from which to choose: jogging, cycling, rowing, stair climbing, walking, swimming, jumping rope, to name just a few. Exercise so that you're breathing hard but can still carry on a labored conversation. The harder, the better.

To continue making gains, you should incorporate fascial stretching into your workouts. Fascial stretching elicits responses in muscle groups that have reached sticking points in training. If you have a certain muscle that still seems at a stalemate in size, strength, or appearance, stretching it will help you overcome these frustrating plateaus.

49 AVOID LAYOFFS AND MAKE GREATER PROGRESS

You may have read somewhere that your favorite bodybuilder takes a layoff from training every several months, usually to restore mental and physical energy. In my opinion, layoffs aren't a good idea, unless you're ill or need to recuperate from an injury.

By not working out for a period of time, you lose a lot of ground. Your muscle shrinks, so you lose size and tone. Not only that, your ability to sustain muscular contractions will be weakened due to reduced nerve fiber stimulation in the muscles. The nerves therefore can't adequately discharge motor impulses to the working muscles. As a result, you're able to complete fewer reps with less weight. Strength definitely suffers.

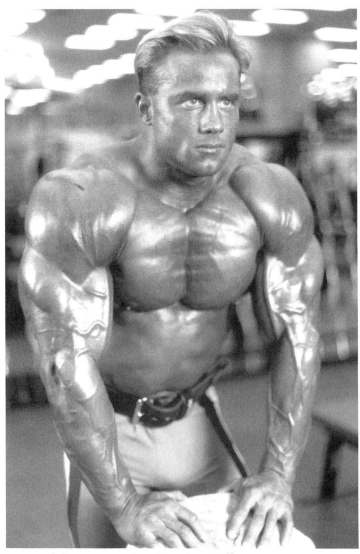

Intensity is the name of the game. *Photo by Irvin J. Gelb.*

My advice is to never slack off. And when you're in the gym, aim for new poundage levels and more intensity each workout. Always enter the gym with this attitude: "Today will be my best workout ever." Some bodybuilders, however, advocate heavy, medium, and light days. This could hold you back. If you're fueling yourself properly with the right foods and nutritional supplements, your lifts and your intensity should continually increase.

But what if you pick up a particular weight and it feels heavy? This may be an indication that you haven't fully recovered from a previous workout. That being so, pump out as many reps as you can, just to get the blood moving through the muscles. This delivers more nutrients to muscle cells, hastening recovery.

Sure, you'll have good days and bad days in the gym. Everyone does. If you have a bad day, try to figure out why. After all, no one knows your body better than you do.

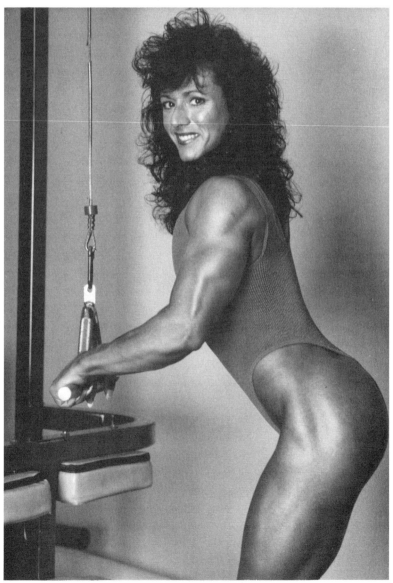

During the negative portion of the exercise, use the strength of your biceps to return the weight to the starting position, as Dona Oliveira demonstrates. *Photo by Jimmie D. King.*

50 MENTAL ACUITY: GET PSYCHED TO GET RESULTS

Three factors go into building a great physique: proper nutrition, intense training, and mental acuity. Proper nutrition is the foundation, supplying the energy you need to train hard and the raw materials for muscular growth. Training provides the stimulus for growth. What makes the first two gel is mental acuity—the commitment and concentration it takes to adhere to the right nutrition and training programs. You're not going to achieve your physique goals if you're splurging every other day on refined carbohydrates and processed foods—or if your mind wanders during your workout, and you quit halfway through.

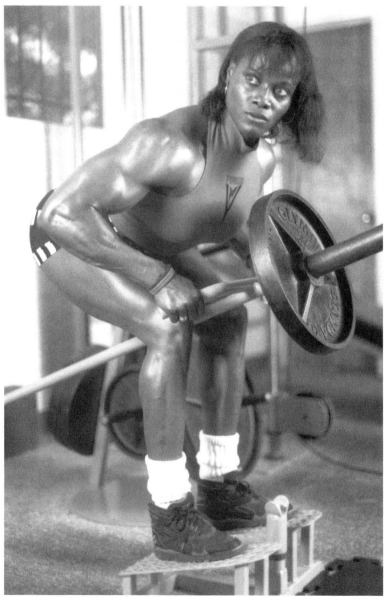

Yolanda Hughes concentrates intensely on perfect form when training her back. *Photo by Irvin J. Gelb.*

How do you sharpen your mental acuity? In seven ways, as I see it:

- *Energy.* Fulfilling your daily energy requirements with ample calories and nutrients is so critical that it bears repeating. After all, you won't be able to withstand a hard workout—or recover from that workout—if you're not consuming a high-nutrient-density diet. Good nutrition shores up your mental energy, too. You'll feel better and have a more positive outlook.
- *Self-assessment.* Be able to assess yourself honestly. This includes your diet, your training program, and your progress. Does your diet measure up in terms of calories, nutrients, and food choices? Equally important is consistency. Are you staying on course? The same questions can be applied to training. Analyze your exercises to see whether you're challenging yourself to do more each workout.
- *Avoid comparisons.* Don't fall into the trap of comparing yourself to others. You're unique, with the ability to become the best you are or to perform to your own distinct potential. If you find yourself comparing your physique to the physiques of elite bodybuilders and athletes, use that comparison as a general standard of what can be achieved by nutrition, training, and dedication.
- *Concentration.* You must never let your mind wander while you're working out. The pressures of everyday life have a way of letting themselves through the gym door. Fight this intrusion at all costs by focusing on the present—each rep, each set, each exercise.
- *Balance.* Dedication to bodybuilding is integral to high-level success. But if your focus is too narrow—that is, if you pursue bodybuilding to the exclusion of relationships, hobbies, and your career, for example—then you're skewing your perspective on life. Have balance in your life, with a range of experiences that contributes to your personal growth. You'll be a better bodybuilder as a result.
- *Have a road map.* You can make progress much faster if you know the direction. Map out your diet—for the day, the week, and the month—making adjustments in your caloric levels according to the changes in your physique. Follow a written training routine and keep records of your reps, sets, and poundages. The point is to exceed your previous levels of effort.
- *Believe in yourself.* You may have all the support in the world, but success comes down to one thing: belief in yourself. I've never seen bodybuilders achieve their goals if they didn't believe they could. Don't just *hope* you can get there—*believe* you can.

The choice to form positive new habits in training and in life is yours alone to make. If you want to move closer to your goals and achieve those things that make you happy, then make choices that are best for your personal health and well-being.

The most important thing you can do in life is to live up to your potential. You have to believe in yourself and take steps to reach that potential.

In every moment that passes, continue to practice discipline, take responsibility, and enjoy your accomplishments. For these are the experiences that will give you the confidence to succeed in whatever you do.

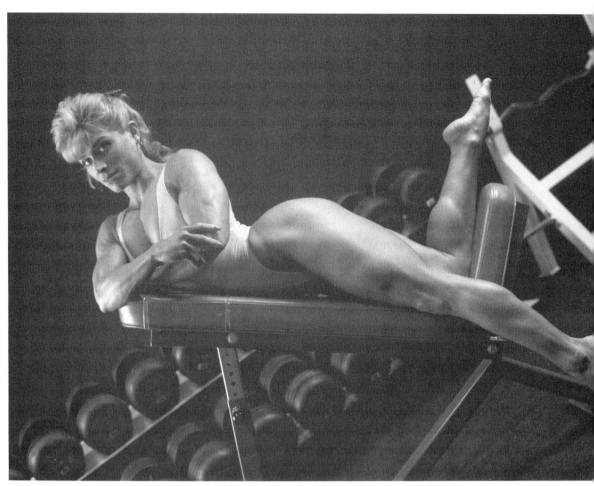

Mental acuity is the commitment and concentration it takes to get results like these. *Photo by Ralph DeHaan.*

Appendix

BODYSTAT CHARTING

Building lean muscle is the major goal of any bodybuilding program. To measure your progress toward that goal, you must check your body composition, preferably on a weekly basis. BodyStat Charting is a system I developed for monitoring muscle-to-fat ratios. It uses skinfold calipers, the most accurate testing method for people below 15 percent body fat, and applies special calculations to give you an accurate assessment of your ratio of body weight to body fat, percentage of body fat, pounds of body fat, and pounds of muscle mass.

A skinfold caliper device measures the thickness of a fold of skin with its underlying layer of fat. Skinfold calipers have springs that exert pressure on the skinfold and an accurate scale that measures the thickness in millimeters. Because of the locations of these skinfolds, you can't measure yourself. Another person must take your measurements.

Place the jaws of the caliper on the skinfold. The jaws should be about ¼ inch from the fingers of your left hand. Completely release the trigger of the caliper so that the entire force of the jaws is on the skinfold. Don't release the fingers of your left hand while you take the readings.

The jaws will slide slightly to a lower reading as they are first applied. This happens because interstitial fluid is being squeezed from the skin. In seconds, the sliding will stop. At this point, the reading on the scale of the calipers should be read and recorded.

Skinfolds are measured at nine strategic locations on the body:

1. Pec. Measure about one inch below the collarbone and three to four inches out from the inside edge of the pectoral muscle. If you're measuring a woman, be sure to stay on the pec and avoid breast tissue. Pull the skinfold in a horizontal direction.

2. Subscapular. Locate the middle of the scapula (shoulder blade) and measure about one inch in toward the spine. Pull the skinfold in a vertical direction.

3. Biceps. Measure in the middle of the biceps muscle. Pull the skinfold in a vertical direction.

4. Triceps. Measure at the bottom of the inside triceps head. Pull the skinfold in a vertical direction.

5. Kidney. Locate the dimple or indentation above the gluteal muscles. Go up about two inches and out about two inches. Pull the skinfold in a horizontal direction.

6. Suprailiac. Measure about halfway between the navel and the top of the hip bone. This should be at or near the area where the obliques and abdominals meet. Pull the skinfold in a horizontal direction.

7. Abdominals. Measure about one inch to the left of the navel, or one inch to the right, and one inch down. Pull the skinfold in a vertical direction.

8. Quadriceps. Measure in the middle of the quadriceps. If the area is too tight, move up one or two inches to get a reading. Pull the skinfold in a vertical direction.

9. Medial calf. Measure the middle of the inside head. If that area is too tight, move up one or two inches. Pull the skinfold in a vertical direction.

HOW TO INTERPRET THE NUMBERS

After recording the nine measurements, make the following calculations to determine your body composition:

1. Add the nine measurements and divide the total by your body weight. This figure gives you the ratio of body fat to body weight.

2. Multiply that ratio by .27 to get your percentage of body fat.

3. Multiply your percentage of body fat by your body weight to yield your pounds of body fat.

4. Subtract the pounds of body fat from your total body weight to calculate the pounds of lean mass.

Here's an example to illustrate how these calculations work:

1. After adding your nine BodyStat Charting measurements, you get a total of 65. Divide 65 by your body weight (200) to get a body fat to body weight ratio of .32.

2. Multiply your body weight to body fat ratio (.32) by .27 to get a body fat percentage of 8%.

3. Multiply your body weight (200) by your percentage of body fat (8%) to get 16 pounds of body fat.

4. Subtract the pounds of body fat (16) from your body weight (200) to get your total lean muscle mass of 184 pounds.

Notes

Introduction

1. J. Nutter, "Physical increases bone density," NSCA *Journal* 8: 67–69, 1986.

4: The Truth about Fructose

1. D. L. Costill et al., "The role of dietary carbohydrates in muscle glycogen re-synthesis after strenuous running," *American Journal of Clinical Nutrition* 34: 1831–36, 1981.

5: Protein and Muscular Hardness

1. I. Celejowa and M. Homa, "Food intake, nitrogen, and energy balance in Polish weight lifters during training camp," *Nutrition Metabolism* 12: 259–74, 1970.

2. P. W. R. Lemon et al., "Effect of dietary protein and body building exercise on muscle mass and strength gains," *Canadian Journal of Sports Science* 15: 14, 1990. Also: M. A. Tarnopolsky et al., "Effect of body building exercise on protein requirements," *Canadian Journal of Sports Science* 15: 22, 1990.

6: The Energy to Train All Out

1. J. Bergstrom et al., "Diet, muscle glycogen and physical performance," *Acta Physiology Scandinavian* 71: 140–50, 1967.

7: Supplemental Nutrition for Aerobic Energy

1. E. Haymes, "Proteins, vitamins, and iron," in *Ergogenic Aids in Sport*, ed. M. H. Williams (Human Kinetics Publishers, 1983), pp. 27–55. Also: N. S. Scrimshaw, "Iron deficiency," *Scientific American*, pp. 46–52, Oct. 1991.

2. Haymes, "Proteins, vitamins, and iron."

9: Supercompensation

1. D. R. Lamb, A. C. Snyder, and T. S. Baur, "Muscle glycogen loading with a liquid carbohydrate supplement," *International Journal of Sport Nutrition* 1: 52–60, 1991.

12: Train Your Muscles to Burn More Fat

1. E. Jansson et al., "Changes in muscle fiber type distribution in man," *Acta Physiology Scandinavian* 104: 235–37, 1978.

13: Regulating Growth by Exercise and Nutrition

1. D. M. Crist, *Growth Hormone Synergism* (Albuquerque, N.M.: DMC Health Sciences, 1991).

About the Authors

John Parrillo

Nutrition and training expert John Parrillo is the author of *High Performance Bodybuilding*, which describes his revolutionary bodybuilding program of high-calorie nutrition, supplementation, fascial stretching, special training techniques, and body composition charting.

Mr. Parrillo has been described by a leading bodybuilding magazine as "an exercise and nutrition genius who knows more about maximizing muscle growth and losing body fat than anyone else in the world."

A former powerlifter and bodybuilder, he has worked with professional and amateur bodybuilders, powerlifters, endurance athletes, pro wrestlers, and other athletes for twenty years, teaching them how to diet and train for maximum performance and results.

Mr. Parrillo is the author of several manuals on his programs. In addition, he writes nutrition and training articles for various magazines and is a columnist for *MuscleMag International*, *Muscle Training Illustrated*, *Ironman*, and *American Fitness Quarterly*. He publishes his own magazine, *John Parrillo's Performance Press*, from the Parrillo Performance offices in Cincinnati, Ohio.

Maggie Greenwood-Robinson

In addition to *John Parrillo's 50 Workout Secrets*, Maggie Greenwood-Robinson is the coauthor of three other fine books: BUILT! *The New Bodybuilding for Everyone* (with Robert Kennedy), *Cliff Sheats' Lean Bodies* (with Cliff Sheats), and *High Performance Bodybuilding* (with John Parrillo).

Ms. Greenwood-Robinson writes a regular column on weight training for *Female Bodybuilding*, as well as articles for other fitness magazines. Her articles have included such topics as weight training during pregnancy, strength training for sports, body sculpting, nutritional supplementation, and high-tech fitness. Ms. Greenwood-Robinson's articles have appeared in *American Health*, *Muscle & Fitness*, *Ironman*, *Female Bodybuilding*, *MuscleMag International*, *Bodybuilding Lifestyles*, *Work Out*, and other magazines.

Get fit with the best names in physical fitness and strength training.

These books are available at your bookstore or wherever books are sold, or, for your convenience, we'll send them directly to you. Call 1-800-631-8571 (press 1 for inquiries and orders) or fill out the coupon below and send it to:

The Berkley Publishing Group
390 Murray Hill Parkway, Department B
East Rutherford, NJ 07073

	ISBN	U.S.	CAN
____ *Sports Strength* by Ken Sprague	399-51802-9	$16.95	$22.50
____ *The Gold's Gym Book of Weight Training* by Ken Sprague	399-51846-0	$14.00	$18.50
____ *Weight and Strength Training for Kids and Teenagers* by Ken Sprague	874-77643-0	$12.95	
____ *Gold's Gym Book of Strength Training* by Ken Sprague	399-51863-0	$14.00	$18.50
____ *High-Performance Bodybuilding* by John Parrillo and Maggie Greenwood-Robinson	399-51771-5	$16.00	$21.00
____ *Big* by Ellington Darden, Ph.D.	399-51630-1	$16.00	$21.00
____ *Bigger Muscles in 42 Days* by Ellington Darden, Ph.D.	399-51706-5	$16.00	$21.00
____ *High-Intensity Strength Training* by Ellington Darden, Ph.D.	399-51770-7	$16.00	$21.00
____ *Massive Muscles in 10 Weeks* by Ellington Darden, Ph.D.	399-51340-X	$16.00	$21.00
____ *New High-Intensity Bodybuilding* by Ellington Darden, Ph.D.	399-51614-X	$15.95	$20.95
____ *The Six-Week Fat-to-Muscle Makeover* by Ellington Darden, Ph.D.	399-51562-3	$9.95	$12.95
____ *High-Intensity Home Training* by Ellington Darden, Ph.D.	399-51840-1	$15.95	$20.95
____ *John Parrillo's 50 Workout Secrets* by John Parrillo and Maggie Greenwood-Robinson (Available July 1994)	399-51862-2	$16.00	$21.00

Subtotal $ _____
Postage & handling* $ _____
Sales tax (CA, NY, NJ, PA) $ _____
Total amount due $ _____
Payable in U.S. funds (no cash orders accepted).
$15.00 minimum for credit card orders.

*Postage & handling: $2.50 for 1 book, 75¢ each additional book up to a maximum of $6.25.

Enclosed is my ☐ check ☐ money order
Please charge my ☐ Visa ☐ Mastercard ☐ American Express

Card #_____ Expiration date _____

Signature as on charge card _____

Name _____

Address _____

City _____ State _____ Zip _____
Please allow six weeks for delivery. Prices subject to change without notice.

69